Hell...
be difficult, too....

Don't be surprised if your baby, toddler, or pre-schooler is distant, irritable, or downright angry at you when you reunite at the end of your workday. Giving you the cold shoulder or acting out is often a child's way of letting you know that he's not happy you left him in the first place, and is typical of behavior during the first few weeks of your returning to work and leaving him or her in someone else's care. Some children even refuse to go to their parents when they arrive; they may busy themselves with an activity and ignore you. No matter how much you may have anticipated sweeping your child up in your arms and getting a big hug and kiss, don't let your disappointment interfere with your actions. Take cues from the daycare provider or sitter (who should help the child with your return). Or give your child a few minutes to say hello again. You might make some ordinary conversation, such as asking your child what kind of structure he's building or compliment her on the beautiful pictures she's painting. . . .

Also from the editors of *Child* magazine

Sleep: How to Teach Your Child to Sleep Like a Baby
Tantrums: Secrets to Calming the Storm

Published by POCKET BOOKS

From the Editors of **child** Magazine

GOODBYES

how to say
"see you later" to your
little alligator

Nancy Hall and Peggy Schmidt

A New Century Communications Book

POCKET BOOKS
New York   London   Toronto   Sydney   Tokyo   Singapore

The author of this book is not a physician and the ideas, procedures, and suggestions in this book are not intended as a substitute for the medical advice of a trained health professional. All matters regarding your child's health require medical supervision. Consult your child's physician before adopting the suggestions in this book, as well as about any condition that may require diagnosis or medical attention. The author and publisher disclaim any liability arising directly or indirectly from the use of the book.

An *Original* Publication of POCKET BOOKS

POCKET BOOKS, a division of Simon & Schuster Inc.
1230 Avenue of the Americas, New York, NY 10020

Copyright © 1996 by Peggy Schmidt

ISBN: 0-671-88037-3

First Pocket Books printing July 1996

10 9 8 7 6 5 4 3 2 1

POCKET and colophon are registered trademarks of Simon & Schuster Inc.

Cover photo by Tosca Radigonda Felicello

Printed in the U.S.A.

For Wilson and Margaret, and for David
—Nancy Hall

For my daughter Christina and my son Ted
—Peggy Schmidt

Acknowledgments

Our deepest appreciation to the following people who shared their expertise with us:

Jay Belsky, Ph.D., professor of human development at Pennsylvania State University, University Park, Pennsylvania

Martha Cox, Ph.D., research professor at the University of North Carolina at Chapel Hill

Frank Dobisky, president, Dobisky & Associates, Keene, New Hampshire

Byron Egeland, Ph.D., professor of child development at the University of Minnesota, Minneapolis, Minnesota

Martha Farrell Erickson, Ph.D., director of the University of Minnesota's Children, Youth, and Family Consortium, Minneapolis, Minnesota

Tiffany Field, Ph.D., a professor in the University of Miami Medical School's departments of Pediatrics, Psychology, and Psychiatry, Miami, Florida

Linda Goudas, Ph.D., staff psychologist at Children's Hospital, Boston, Massachusetts

Alicia Lieberman, Ph.D., professor of psychology at the University of California, San Francisco, California

Merle Marsh, head of the Lower and Middle Schools, Worcester Country School, Franford, Maryland

Kathleen McCue, M.A., L.S.W., supervisor of the Child Life Program at the Cleveland Clinic Foundation and president of the National Child Life Council, Cleveland, Ohio

Marilyn Montgomery, Ph.D., founder of the Wellspring Center for Family Development, Lubbock, Texas

Frederic J. Medway, Ph.D., professor of psychology at the University of South Carolina, Columbia, South Carolina

M. G. Mendes de Leon, coordinator of the Child Life Program at Yale–New Haven Hospital, New Haven, Connecticut

Kathy Nathan, Ph.D., director of the Child Development Research Center at Texas Tech University, Lubbock, Texas

Stana Paulauskas, Ph.D., clinical child psychologist at Ohio State University Psychiatric Health Care, Columbus, Ohio

William Pfohl, Psy.D., professor of psychology at Western Kentucky University, Bowling Green, Kentucky

Janine Wenzel Reed, Ph.D., clinical psychologist in private practice, Los Altos, California

Leslie Rescorla, Ph.D., associate professor of psychology at Bryn Mawr College, Bryn Mawr, Pennsylvania

Julia Robertson, M.D., assistant professor, University of Louisville School of Medicine, Department of Psychiatry, Louisville, Kentucky

Patricia Schindler, director of Newcomb Children's Center of Tulane University, New Orleans, Louisiana

Carol Seefeldt, Ph.D., professor of human development at the Institute for Child Study, University of Maryland, College Park, Maryland

Barbara Talent, Ph.D., clinical psychologist with the Child Development Center at St. John's Mercy Hospital, St. Louis, Missouri

Marsha Weinraub, Ph.D., professor of psychology at Temple University, Philadelphia, Pennsylvania

Contents

Letter from the Editor

Dear Reader:

Expectant parents are quick to fill their shelves with books to prepare them for what's to come. But once the baby arrives, moms and dads are more likely to turn to information that's accessible, to the point, and a quick read. We created the *Child* Magazine Series for Parents for just that reason.

What makes the *Child* Magazine Series for Parents unique is that each book is intended to help parents of young children—babies, toddlers, preschoolers, and early school-age children—deal with a specific problem—quickly. The books are written by accomplished journalists who have picked the brains of leading child psychologists, researchers, and child-care experts and organized their collective wisdom. The benefit to you is that you will be presented with a number of strategies for understanding and coping with your child's behavior. You can select the one that best suits your parenting style, or try more than one if the first one you choose doesn't achieve the change you're looking for.

If you're a busy parent who needs help *now* to solve the problem featured in this book, I hope you will pick it up and start reading it tonight. I'm sure that the small investment of your time will provide a quick return as you implement the solutions we present. Throughout the book, you will find age "flags" that will help you easily find the sections that relate most directly to your situation. And if you find this advice helpful, try another book in this series; each one is written in the same friendly, informative style as *Child* magazine articles.

We'd love to hear from you after you have read the book. Let us know what worked for you, and whether you have any additional ideas that we might include in future editions of this book. Write to us at: *Child, Child* Magazine Series for Parents, 110 Fifth Avenue, New York, NY 10003. Or e-mail us at: Childmag@aol.com.

Pamela Abrams
Editor-in-Chief

Introduction

Why "Good" Goodbyes Are So Important

When it came time for me to go back to work, I thought that saying goodbye to my baby would be a piece of cake. I had studied daycare and parent–child separations for a living as a doctoral candidate in a child development program at Yale University. I knew what to look for, what to avoid, what my options were. I had connections. I had resources. I knew my baby and I would both survive this separation, and even flourish if I did it right.

Why then, in spite of everything I knew about the need to allow plenty of time and do all my research, did I find myself putting off making arrangements for this separation until just a few weeks before I had to be back at the office? Every time I thought about making the first list of people to call or centers to visit or babysitters to interview, something important always came up instead—something like taking our amazing new son to the park or simply sitting with him and nuzzling the back of his perfect neck.

In the end, I handled this separation the way most people do—reluctantly and relying on my gut instincts. When our next-door neighbor told me that the woman who looked after her 6-month-old in the mornings was interested in taking another child as well, we signed up. When my son was 3 months old and I left him there for a few hours on the first day, he beamed his blithe baby smile at the caregiver as I left, and I sobbed the 30 miles to work.

I knew I wanted to continue with my work and my studies, but every fiber of my newly sprung maternal being bristled and quivered as I pulled away from the caregiver's door that day. Why, I kept asking, why do we have to do it this way? Why do we have to be apart? Why can't I just strap him to my back and keep right on going?

That same son is 6 years old now, a happy, bright, kind little boy who separates easily from me and his dad for school or baseball or a friend's birthday party. But he still loves to curl up with us for a story or some comfort when he's sick or sometimes just for a good snuggle. Only now am I sure that I did the right thing in continuing with my work. But until I had done it myself, all the study and research in the world couldn't have convinced me how agonizing such separations are, nor would I have understood their value.

Never before have parents and children routinely separated so early, so often, or for such long periods of time. Almost 60 percent of mothers with children under the age of 6 work, usually full time. And most parents have friends, neighbors, relatives, and babysitters care for their young children so they can take care of the business of daily life or have an occasional night or weekend to themselves.

Whether you work outside the home or care for your child full time (or your spouse does), separations are inevitable. Avoiding separations doesn't do you or your child any good in the long run—they are a fact of modern life, and learning to handle them is an important step along the road to self-reliance and maturity. The greatest gift you can give your child is the capacity to not only weather separations, but to learn from them. Children who are able to do this will be well equipped to balance independence and closeness throughout their lives.

The advantages of separation for your child may not appear immediately obvious when she is wailing about being left with a sitter, but over time you will realize that there are many benefits for her, including:

- Enlarging her world and bringing her new experiences
- Making room for other people in your child's life. Even very young children delight in having special grown-up friends who care for them, and being in the company of children their own age is important even to very young children.
- Providing invaluable practice for the days when your child heads off to nursery school, kindergarten, and first grade
- Helping your child develop a greater sense of independence and self-reliance. Being reunited with you again after brief separations enhances his sense of trust in you.

Separation involves much more than learning to overcome your initial reluctance at returning to work after childbirth or adoption, or getting your baby through the throes of stranger anxiety at 8 or 9 months of age. The first separation of the infant from the mother is probably the most difficult—at least for the mother—but the skills learned by both of you will lay the groundwork for helping the child deal with everything from her first playdate with a toddler friend to adjusting to day care or nursery school to dealing with the death of a pet or having a best friend move away during grade school.

Separation concerns don't end with childhood, either. Adults are asked to say goodbye, too; romances end, friends move, children go away to college, and loved ones die. The separation process is lifelong, but much of what sets the stage for success occurs between infancy and 5 years of age. The way we were taught to deal with separation early in our lives will color the way we handle these events.

As a parent, you probably truly love spending time with your child, but you, too, can also benefit from time spent apart. In fact, having some time of your own is essential for holding a job, getting chores done, and maintaining some sense of your own identity beyond your role as a parent. Your relationship with your spouse or partner is enhanced when you have child-free time. Although it may seem ironic, having time to attend to your own needs is likely to make you more responsive to the needs of your child.

Since separations from your child are inevitable, it is important to prepare your child and yourself for them. What works to help infants deal with separations may not be appropriate for preschool children, and the issues faced by a 3-year-old going off to daycare will be different from the concerns you have about an 18-month-old child who follows you incessantly from room to room. Children react differently depending on their age, developmental level, and temperament. Situations differ, too; you will have one set of concerns about going out several times a month with your spouse and others about taking a 5-day business trip. Some separations, like dropping your child off at a daycare, are routine, while others, like hospitalizations (for parent or child) are more precipitous and potentially traumatic.

In the pages that follow, you will learn what to expect as you and your child part at different ages. You'll learn what the experts have to say and how parents like you have weathered difficult goodbyes and learned from them. The chapters are arranged to help you easily locate topics and situations that interest you most. Chapter One starts with the basics of what separations are all about and how you can take advantage of your child's unique personality to guide you through them successfully. Chapter Two is devoted to the concerns of women who plan to return to work when their maternity leave is up or at a later time before their child starts school. Chapter Three is a guide for negotiating that most difficult of getaways—an evening out! Chapter Four covers making the transition into preschool and kindergarten—not just the big goodbye in September, but subsequent parting problems that may arise as your child goes through developmental changes and stresses. Chapter Five deals with the longer parental absences because of business trips and vacations (yes, you should take them!). And Chapter Six offers advice on coping with more traumatic goodbyes that are precipitated by military duty, illness, or family relocations.

Sections within each chapter are flagged so that you can readily see whether a particular section applies to your child. There are also strategies for dealing with bad goodbye behavior and techniques on how to prepare your child for specific separations. In addition, a Resource section at the end of this book lists books, articles, and agencies to contact for additional information on topics in this book.

NOTE: When the first person is used in this book, it refers to Nancy Hall.

🌀 ONE

Saying Hello to Goodbyes

Separations from your child are as much a part of your everyday world and your child's as the cuddles and closeness you share. And learning to be apart from each other from time to time is important. Whether you are putting your child in her playpen for 15 minutes so you can shower and dress, leaving her with a trusted sitter while you have an evening out, or saying goodbye at the daycare center door on your way to work, separations big and small are an inevitable part of the lives of young children.

That being the case, you will be doing yourself and your child a service if you teach your child to handle goodbyes with ease. Children who are able to comfortably leave their parents' side will be well equipped to balance independence and closeness with their parents and other loved ones throughout their lives. "It's normal and healthy for a child to sometimes show unhap-

1

piness when you say goodbye to each other," says Martha Cox, Ph.D., research professor at the University of North Carolina at Chapel Hill. "It's also important for you to acknowledge the unhappiness by saying something like 'You'll miss me, and I'll miss you, but I'm glad you can have fun while I'm gone.'"

Even though leaving your baby, toddler, or preschooler in the care of others may be difficult for you, you cannot afford to let your anxiety interfere with modeling good goodbye behavior. "How you cope with separation will play a big role in how your child deals with it," says Stana Paulauskas, Ph.D., clinical assistant professor of psychiatry at Ohio State University. "If you avoid it or act overly concerned about leaving your child, she will learn that you are scared about separations and will learn to fear them, too," she adds.

Psychologists often talk about separation anxiety in relation to two concepts: dependence and attachment. John Bowlby, M.D., a pioneer in the research of separation on the development of the child, notes in his classic *Separation: Anxiety and Anger,* that an infant's state of helplessness (dependence) is at its greatest at birth and diminishes as the child matures and becomes independent, while attachment (the strong emotional bond between parent and child) is absent at birth but becomes apparent at about 6 months of age. It is a secure attachment that allows a child to develop his "wings"—that is, the self-confidence to try new situations and new people on his own and become an independent person.

It's easy to think that those wings may never sprout if your child wails uncontrollably, kicks, or screams when you leave. You can quickly lose your resolve to go out and have a good time or plan product strategy for a client meeting later in the morning. But if you realize that goodbyes are harder for children with particular types of temperaments and at different stages of development, you will become more skilled at making them an opportunity for growth and change for both you and your child.

Of course, there are also goodbye crises that can occur without warning, just when you and your child have both settled comfortably into an easy routine of nursery school drop-offs, going out on regular dates with your spouse, or having a sitter in a few hours a day while you exercise and run errands. It's normal for most children 6 and under to occasionally have trouble leaving their parents' side at one time or another. Sometimes difficult goodbyes are the result of stress the child is feeling because of changes in her routine or her world, or they may result from developmental phases your child is undergoing.

THE ROLE OF TEMPERAMENT

Child psychologists say the single biggest determinant of whether your child will have problems with goodbyes over time is her temperament. "Some kids are flexible; others are routine oriented," explains Leslie Rescorla, Ph.D., associate professor in the department of psychology at Bryn Mawr College in Pennsylvania. "Those who are more easy-going and can roll with the punches are going to have an easier time being away from their parents. The child who is slow to warm up to new kids and adults and who functions best with minimal change is going to have a tougher time," she says.

Just what is temperament? Psychiatrists Stella Chess, M.D., and Alexander Thomas, M.D., and behavioral scientist Herbert Birch, M.D., were able to identify nine temperament traits through a study that began in the mid-1950s and is still ongoing. Many experts now agree that children are born with these behavioral preferences. While none are inherently good or bad, whether your child rates low or high on certain of these traits can affect whether he has a hard time with goodbyes. Toward the end of your child's first year, if not sooner, you should be able to detect patterns in his behavioral style. Where does your child fall on each of these scales?

1. *Activity Level*—the amount of physical movement a child performs and the proportion of active to inactive periods per day. Examples:

    High activity—a baby who waves her arms, rolls her head, and wiggles a lot; a preschooler who is always on the go and physically active

    Low activity—a baby who sits or lays quietly in his stroller; a preschooler who prefers quiet play activities to noisy, physical ones

2. *Regularity (or rhythmicity)*—the predictability (or unpredictability) of a child's daily patterns of eating, sleeping, and defecating. Examples:

> *High regularity*—a baby who gets tired and goes down for naps at the same times every day; a preschooler who sleeps 12 hours every night

> *Low regularity*—an infant whose eating needs and schedule seem to vary day by day; a preschooler who has bowel movements at different times each day

3. *Approach/withdrawal*—how a child initially responds to a new situation, food, toy, person, place, or other stimulus. Examples:

> *High approach*—a baby who readily picks up and examines a new toy; a preschooler who easily befriends children in a playground

> *High withdrawal*—a baby who refuses to leave a mother's lap or side when they go to a play group; a preschooler who is reluctant to stay at school if a substitute teacher is in for the day

4. *Adaptability*—how easily a child adapts to a new or altered situation over time. Examples:

> *High adaptability*—a baby who has no trouble falling asleep when her bassinet is replaced by a crib; a preschooler who adjusts to a new, permanent sitter after spending a short time with her

> *Low adaptability*—a baby who cries and squirms every time you put her in a carseat; a preschooler who prefers his worn-at-the-knee pants to new clothing

5. *Sensory threshold*—the point at which any given stimulus will evoke a response from the child. Examples:

> *High threshold*—a toddler who falls down while running and just gets back up; a preschooler who can concentrate on a task despite a high level of household noise

> *Low threshold*—a baby who refuses to drink a formula different than what she's accustomed to; a preschooler who cannot fall asleep unless his night light is on and the room is quiet

6. *Intensity*—how forcefully a child expresses his reactions, whether positive or negative. Examples:

> *High intensity*—a baby who wails loudly and long when confined to a playpen; a preschooler whose voice quivers with rage when she's angry, even over small things

> *Low intensity*—a baby who whimpers when frustrated at being unable to make a toy work; a preschooler who frowns or leaves the room when an older sibling teases her relentlessly

7. *Distractibility*—how well the child can pay attention and how easily she is distracted. Examples:

> *High distractibility*—a baby who will stop sucking on his bottle if he hears an unusual noise; a preschooler who stops working on her art proj-

ect frequently in response to other children talking and moving around the classroom.

Low distractibility—an infant who doesn't miss a bite of the dinner being fed him, even when Daddy or Mommy walks in the door after a day at work; a preschooler who cannot be cajoled into play by her sitter because she refuses to leave the window until Mommy is out of sight

8. *Persistence/attention span*—the length of time a child can stay engaged with a particular object or activity, even in the face of obstacles and difficulties. Examples:

High persistence/long attention span—a baby who isn't discouraged from trying to open the cupboard doors to get at pots and pans, even though you have firmly "locked" them; a preschooler who insists on working on a puzzle until she gets it all put together

Low persistence/short attention span—a baby who looks at new objects in her crib only a short time before refocusing her attention elsewhere; a preschooler who asks to have a book read to him, but jumps up to play with something else after you've only read a few pages

9. *Quality of Mood*—the child's basic disposition. Examples:

Positive mood—a baby who smiles and gurgles

most of the time; a preschooler who has a smile and hello for every family member each morning

Negative mood—a baby who rarely acts content; a preschooler who frequently complains there's nothing to do

If you understand your child's temperament, you will be better able to understand her reaction to separations and even orchestrate them to minimize bad reactions. Several of these temperament characteristics are especially relevant to separation issues. If your child rates high on rhythmicity, for example, (that is, she functions best with a predictable routine), try to arrange separations so that they do not interfere with her nap or mealtimes. If your child rates low on adaptability, he will need extra time to get used to a new sitter—try having her come early and play while you get ready so that the transition is more gradual. If your baby rates high on persistence/attention span, she will probably cry and watch the door for a longer time after you leave than does a child at the other end of this scale, who is more likely to return to play relatively quickly. If you clue in the sitter to that trait, she won't feel frustrated in her attempts to distract your child and will know to let her come around to accepting your departure.

STAGES THROUGH THE AGES: WHAT TO EXPECT WHEN YOU SAY GOODBYE

Goodbyes are usually a much bigger issue for you than they are for your child during her first 6 months of life. When separation anxiety (a fear of unfamiliar faces)

sets in at around 9 months of age, goodbyes can be painful for both of you. Toddlerhood and the preschool years are punctuated by periods of stress because of the kinds of transitions you're asking your little one to make: going to preschool, having playdates with friends, spending more time with caregivers so that you can take classes, go back to work part time, or enjoy evenings out with your spouse. Here's an age-by-age guide to the challenges of separation from birth to age 6.

Great Beginnings: The First 6 Months

AGE FLAG: BIRTH TO 6 MONTHS

Before your baby can learn to separate from you, he first has to learn to be close to you. Everything about the human baby is geared to keeping him close to those who will love and protect him. His vision at birth, for instance, is clearest for objects about 12 inches away, just the distance of your face from his while you feed him. Infants also display a preference for their mothers' voices over those of strangers within about a month of birth. They can tell one caregiver from another, and show a strong preference for those whose caregiving style is sensitive and responsive.

These are ways that your baby is uniquely prepared—programmed, you might almost say—to expect sameness and continuity in her life. These capacities allow you and your baby to become familiar and comfortable with each other very early in your baby's life. "All these very early abilities are used in the service of anticipating what is going to happen next, on the basis of what has happened before. From the very beginning, the mother and the baby are engaged in a sense of rhythm with each other," explains Alicia Lieberman, Ph.D., professor of psychology at the University of California at San Francisco. Your baby will soon come to identify you as the most important person in his life.

THE CONCEPT OF ATTACHMENT

It is this very closeness of the baby to her caregiver (or caregivers) that serves as the basis for healthy separations. The key to virtually all of her later behavior is her developing understanding that the world is a safe, predictable place. For the baby, this means knowing that her needs will be understood and met within a reasonable amount of time by someone she knows and trusts.

Psychologists call this understanding attachment. Research by child-development experts shows that caregiver responsiveness to a baby is the key to healthy attachment. An infant who is securely attached, for instance, will use behaviors like crying to bring a parent near to relieve her distress, and then will be comforted by the parent's holding, cuddling, and caregiving. A secure sense of attachment is vital to healthy and trouble-free separations both in infancy and in later life.

Developing a secure attachment to her caregivers is the baby's most important task during the first year of life, a task that she begins to practice from the earliest days of her life. A baby whose needs are not regularly met, or who has not had the opportunity to become attached to one or two regular caregivers, cannot develop a sense of trust in the continuity and stability of his world. "If a mother is under stress and focused more on her own need, she and her baby will not be able to establish the kind of synchronous exchange that leads to a secure, attached relationship," says Jay Belsky, Ph.D., professor of human development at Pennsylvania State University in University Park. This baby may cry for his mother or caregiver but fail to be completely comforted if she delays getting to him or giving him the right kind of reassurance. Such a baby may well have difficulty with goodbyes later in childhood because he did not form strong attachments to his primary caregivers as an infant.

MOMMY: PRISONER OF LOVE

AGE FLAG: INFANCY TO 6 MONTHS

Babies quickly come to understand who their primary caregiver is. By about 4 months of age, the typical infant will smile more readily for her mother (or father, if he is the primary caregiver) than for anyone else.

Continuity of care—arranging a reasonably predictable routine for your baby in which she is cared for in the same way every day—is important, say child-development experts. If the mother believes that she and *only* she can take care of the baby, however, the baby has no opportunity to learn that her needs can be taken care of by somebody else. When Dad or Grandma or a hired caregiver fill in, as they inevitably will, baby is more likely to be upset because the familiar smell, touch, look, sound, and feel of Mom isn't there. A baby, even a newborn, is quite capable of learning to cope with minor variations in her routine. Sometimes it is Mom who comes to hold and feed her. Sometimes Dad comes and carries her in a front carrier while he prepares her dinner. Sometimes she is handed carefully to her older brother for a cuddle or to her grandmother or her uncle for a diapering or a bath.

Just as there is a down side if no one but Mom cares for her baby, there is a disadvantage to having too many caregivers. If you have arranged for a patchwork quilt of people to take care of your new son (if you must return to work right away, for example), he will be unable to predict who will be taking care of his needs, and his capacity for trust may well be impaired. This lack of a secure attachment can result in your baby resisting being away from you.

GOODBYES TO BABY PAVE THE WAY

AGE FLAG: NEWBORN TO 6 MONTHS

Is it silly to talk to your infant, when you go out, about where you are going and when you will return? Absolutely not, according to Dr. Lieberman. "First, it creates a habit of communication that then becomes very natural. Even infants 6 months and younger associate your soothing tone of voice, eye contact, and the way you hold them with a predictable and nonthreatening leave-taking," she says. The fact that your baby doesn't understand your words isn't important; what is important is that you are setting up a pattern for goodbyes in the future. You let your baby know that you're going, you kiss her goodbye, and you hand her over to the waiting arms of your spouse or caregiver.

Orchestrating Successful First Goodbyes

AGE FLAG: NEWBORN TO 6 MONTHS

1. Make early separations as stress-free as possible. Plan your time away so that your baby is rested and content; it will make longer separations easier in the coming weeks.

2. Go away for the same few hours each time. Even babies in the first half-year of life benefit from routines that help them to develop a sense that life is predictable and stable.

3. Don't delay your first few outings away from baby. It's normal for separations at this stage to be far tougher on you than on your baby. You may feel a powerful longing to get home quickly the first few times. Or, after looking forward to an outing, you may suddenly find yourself reluctant to leave. Go. You, too, will learn that your baby can be cared for by someone else.

4. Try to use the same caregiver each time; it will be easier for you and your child.

Yikes! A New Face

AGE FLAG: 6 TO 12 MONTHS

Your baby beams and gurgles as the sitter arrives, and you've made it to work every day this month without shedding a tear on the way. You and your spouse are getting out occasionally, leaving baby and sitter equally calm and happy at home. Then one day, usually without warning, things change. Your baby clings to you as you try to drop her off at the family daycare she's been going to all along. Or your mother is offended because her grandchild wails when you try to leave them alone together for an afternoon.

Even if you have mastered the separation issues of the first 6 months, your baby's second 6 months will bring new challenges. When this occurs, rest assured that your baby's development is right on track. In a way, the separation difficulties that typically emerge between 7 and 9 months are a mark of your baby's growing love for you. No one, not her accustomed caregiver, not Grandma, maybe not even Daddy, can hold a candle to Mom at this stage, and your baby is going to let you know this in no uncertain terms.

Your child's sudden reluctance to let you go arises from her growing understanding of how important you are to her. She's also more conscious of unfamiliar people who happen into her universe, a developmental stage that is often called stranger anxiety, but might be thought of more correctly as stranger awareness. Your child has simply come to understand that these people are not you and that they don't measure up for her in the same way you do.

Kathy Nathan, Ph.D., director of Texas Tech University's Child Development Center in Lubbock, assures parents that this is not a bad thing. "Parents should understand that separation anxiety is healthy," she says. "When children are well attached, it's naturally hard to say goodbye."

Stranger awareness typically begins between 7 and 9 months of life, but may persist well into the second year. Separations during this period may be especially challenging, especially if you have to rely on an unfamiliar sitter. And it doesn't matter if that unfamiliar face is a close friend or relative. Your baby may even be initially frightened or shy with his own grandparents if he seldom gets a chance to see them.

Your child is, however, quick to pick up on your feelings, and his response will often mirror yours. If you have mixed emotions about leaving him with a sitter whom you have never before tried, he will pick up on your uneasiness and undoubtedly protest. If, on the other hand, your interactions with the caregiver are congenial and trusting, your baby is likely to warm up to that person too if you give him time. The best strategy is to have a new sitter come for a few trial runs while you're there. There are two benefits: your little one will have an opportunity to slowly get used to a new face, and you have the benefit of being able to judge how adept the sitter is at handling your child.

Your child may still be nonverbal, but now he can understand more of your language. Making verbal goodbyes a part of your separation routine is more important now than ever before. You might use words such as "You'll be here with Mrs. Johnson (or Granddad), and you're going to have a lot of fun while I'm gone." Then leave.

When you and your baby are reunited after a separation, don't be surprised if you get the cold shoulder, at least for the first few minutes you're back in baby's universe. She may avoid making eye contact with you, reaching out for you, or even crawling your way. The reason? It's her way of showing you that she was upset that you were gone. But if you show her how excited you are to see her again through your tone of voice, a gentle physical approach (inviting her into your arms instead of sweeping her up), or by immediately engaging in a game you know she loves, your baby will soon be her affectionate self again.

Out of Sight, Out of Mind?

AGE FLAG: 12 MONTHS TO 2 YEARS

Perhaps the greatest difference between infants and toddlers with respect to separation issues is the toddler's ability to maintain a mental image of you in your absence. Psychologists call this developmental milestone object permanence.

Before your child is in her second year of life, you have probably observed the "out of sight, out of mind" phenomenon occur during play. If she rolled a ball across the living room, she followed it with her eyes until it rolled under the sofa, at which point she appeared to forget about it altogether. For the baby, say psychologists, the ball ceased to exist once she could no longer see it. A toddler, however, would retain an image of the ball in her mind, and if she looked for it without success, she would become distressed if she was unable to retrieve it.

The ability to visualize the ball under the sofa also applies to the parent who has gone into the next room, or to the market, or to work for the day. This new skill is very helpful to your toddler when he is apart from you. The idea that you left yesterday but returned, and did the same thing last week, or the week before, is now much more concrete in your child's mind. Toward the end of his second year, this cognitive capacity is well established, and he is able to use a mental image of you and the understanding that you will come back to comfort himself and enjoy other activities in your absence.

RE-ENACTING GOODBYES AND HELLOS THROUGH GAMES

With their increasing cognitive skills, toddlers are able to use games to act out their parents' departures and returns. This is not just an amusement, but an excellent way of helping them to feel they have some control over these emotionally powerful events.

Have your child play some version of a game in which he hides and then greets a beloved toy again and again. For example, 2-year-old Wilson puts his favorite stuffed bear out in the hallway and says, "Bye-bye," shutting the living-room door firmly behind it. An instant later, he throws the door open and retrieves and hugs his bear. He repeats this behavior again and again. Finally, he flings himself into his mother's lap, yelling, "Hi, Mama!", beaming with pride at his accomplishment. Although the repetitiveness of the activity may drive you crazy, it gives your child a chance to play out separations and reunions. More importantly, he gets to be in charge of them, to control the coming and going of the toy that represents you. Games like peekaboo and "chase me" serve the same function. The delight with which toddlers watch as you hide and uncover your face is derived from their feeling of anticipation and then pleasure as you disappear and then—predictably and safely—return to their view.

A toddler's new mobility brings even more enjoyment to seek-and-find games. Your child runs away from you, then shrieks with delight as you chase and catch him. The thoughts that go through your child's mind are: "I wonder if Daddy will come to get me. I'll bet he'll come to get me. He's coming to get me—hurray!" So bear with your child through the forty-seventh repetition of these goodbye/hello games; when you are reunited at the end of the chase, you both win.

MOBILITY BRINGS INDEPENDENCE AND CLINGINESS

Ironically, the very thing that makes a toddler a toddler—greater physical mobility—turns most children back into clinging vines, at least for a little while. Once your child discovers that he has the power to move away from you, he wants to make sure that this capacity doesn't lead to separations he isn't ready for yet.

When this happens, even children who have happily gone off to spend 1 or 2 hours at a friend's house or parted from you at daycare with no difficulty may suddenly begin to resist letting you go. It may be frustrating to find that you and your child are once again joined at the hip, just as he seemed so much more independent. It can help, though, if you understand that this is your child's way of saying, "I've been off learning to walk, but I'm still yours and I still need to know that you are here when I need you."

This is the next step in a great balancing act—between your child's growing independence and her need to be close to you—that will continue through the preschool and early school years. Although it may seem that you are struggling with separation issues you thought were behind you, the groundwork that you laid during infancy will serve you and your child well now. A child who has begun to develop a strong sense that the world is predictable and trustworthy will weather this stormy period, and so will you.

THE ROLE OF LANGUAGE AND "LOVIES" IN GOODBYES

Toddlers aren't just budding walkers—they're getting to be better talkers, too. You can use your child's growing understanding of language to tie your absence to his daily routine. If you use events in his day to mark when you are going and coming back, particularly routines that he knows well such as mealtime, naptime and playtime, he will be able to more easily grasp what's going to happen. "You'll have your lunch and then your nap, and after your nap I'll be home again" is more meaningful than saying, "I'll be home in 3 hours."

On the other hand, language is becoming a powerful tool in your child's repertoire of behaviors designed to keep you at her side, and this may make goodbyes more difficult. Toddlers have powerful feelings to express, chiefly their love for you, their wish to be near you, and their anger when you go away—however briefly. Language helps them begin to master these strong emotions and to put them into words. Once your child can say "Don't go," he elicits powerful feelings in you, too, especially if you are already ambivalent about leaving. Toddlers are incredibly perceptive about the effect they can have on you, and they are quick to use their growing vocabulary to keep you nearby. Of course, your child may still resort to crying, clinging, or wailing when words fail to achieve the desired effect.

Nevertheless, you cannot afford to be swayed by such manipulations. "Saying goodbye should be a bit hard for both child and parent," says Dr. Kathy Nathan. "The child who shows some distress is a healthy kid because it's indicative of a good bond between parent and child," she says.

Toys and blankets that are special to your child can play an important role in smooth transitions during this period. About half of all young children develop a strong attachment to a "lovy" that she takes with her wherever she goes. The psychological term for a lovy is *transitional object*. And that is exactly what it is—a special tool that helps your child cover the distance from complete dependence on you to greater independence. When you're not there, it offers comfort that can be counted on.

When your child has to leave the security of his home to go to family daycare or his grandparents' house, his special toy or blanket can help him feel more in control of his feelings, and therefore safer and more secure. This inanimate object can also help your child practice the strong emotions of this period. He can fling it down and yell, "I'm mad that you're leaving me," or announce, "I have to go now," without worrying about its reaction. Because lovies can help children express their feelings, you should never discourage him from carrying it around, no matter how dirty or beaten up it gets. Your child will give it up when he is ready, typically before age 4.

You might also try leaving something with your child to remind her that you will be back. It might be a picture of the two of you (encased in a plastic frame) or your sweatshirt.

Establishing Home Base

AGE FLAG: 18 MONTHS TO 3 YEARS

Toddlerhood can best be thought of as a great balancing act among two types of behavior on your child's part, and two types on yours. On her side are the proximity behaviors that have been developing since birth—those behaviors that serve to bring or keep you and your child close together: crying, calling for you, holding onto you, reaching for or running to you, and so on. Exploratory behaviors, on the other hand, are relatively new to the equation. These behaviors help your child practice scouting out and experimenting with her expanding world: walking, running away, ignoring you, reaching for toys. As a parent, you use two corresponding types of behaviors: those aimed at protecting your child (things that bring him closer to you or keep him nearby), and letting-go behaviors that encourage your child to explore his world without being frightened.

When all of these behaviors are in balance, your child can explore his world, then return to you (or another trusted caregiver) to reassure himself that you are still there and he is well protected. When this balance is well established, you serve as what psychologists call a secure home base from which your child can venture for longer and more daring exploration. Healthy separations at this time and for virtually all of the rest of childhood depend on your child's sense that he has such a secure base.

A related hallmark of toddlerhood is the struggle for control, and separation represents a perfect arena for playing out control issues. Your child balks about dressing for daycare, for example—she may even announce that she isn't going at all. If her thriving need for control threatens to get out of hand, defuse some of the power struggle by offering her control over things in which she can have a say. "If you allow your child to make choices about things that are fine for her to control, you reduce the chance of having battles with her on things that are yours, not hers, to decide," says Dr. Nathan. You can't let her decide whether to go to daycare today, or who will care for her while you and your spouse go out for dinner, but she can make choices about smaller things that affect her life. You might ask: "Do you want to take your teddy bear or your rabbit today?" or "Would you like to wear these shorts or your blue sundress when you go to visit Grandma and Grandpa?" Stick to questions that offer a choice, and don't offer an option (the sundress on a cool day, for example) unless you intend to let her select it.

FEARS AND SEPARATION ANXIETY

AGE FLAG: 18 MONTHS TO 3 YEARS

Finally, be aware that children from about 18 months to 3 years of age are prey to a whole host of brand-new fears that may make them unwilling to let you out of their sight. A barking dog, the roaring vacuum cleaner, the dinosaur on television—even a shadow in the dark corner of her bedroom—all appear to present genuine threats requiring your immediate presence. This is perfectly normal, and seems to be connected with the conflicts toddlers feel about closeness and independence, and with not being completely sure they are ready to handle all of their new skills.

Try to balance taking your child's feelings seriously with making her understand that she is in no danger. Sometimes no amount of comfort and hugging from you will completely eliminate these fears—you will just have to pick up your child until the dog stops barking or make sure the night light is placed strategically to eliminate the threatening shadow.

Helping your child to get past her fears will go a long way toward encouraging healthy separations. A child who learns to balance exploration and personal safety is well on the way to feeling independent, competent, and safe.

--------------------- ✳ ---------------------

LEAVING DO'S AND DON'TS

AGE FLAG: 2 YEARS AND UP

Don't apologize for leaving. It conveys the message that you are doing something for which you want your child's forgiveness.

Do treat departures in an upbeat, matter-of-fact way. Say, "I love you and I'll see you after my class today," then give him a hug and kiss and leave. It sends the message that you feel comfortable leaving your child with his caregiver and that he can feel comfortable, too.

Don't ask your child's permission to depart. It gives your child more power than he needs or can comfortably use. Besides, if he responds that it is not all right for you to go, and you go anyway, he will feel (justifiably) that his trust has been violated.

Do say goodbye instead of slipping away. Pulling a disappearing trick may help you avoid a scene today but will jeopardize your child's trust in you, and that will set the stage for more difficult goodbyes in the future.

Don't linger over goodbyes. It shows your ambivalence and may cause your child to feel worried about your leaving, too.

Do talk about what your child will be doing during your separation instead of what you will be doing. Even things you may not consider particularly fun may sound exciting to your youngster. Instead, talk about what she can look forward to doing while you're gone.

Do try to be patient if your toddler acts out when you're reunited. The longer you are gone, the harder it is for her to keep herself together, particularly if she's only 2 or 3. Reunited with you, she feels safe enough to let out a day's worth of emotions all at once. Acknowledge her feelings and tell her how much you missed her.

---- ✳ ----

Preschool and Beyond

AGE FLAG: 3 TO 6 YEARS

The preschool years differ from the toddler years in that preschoolers face many more separation challenges than a toddler, who probably still spends most of his time in your presence or that of a trusted caregiver. The preschool and early school-age child also has a whole collection of new skills and opportunities working in his favor as he broadens his social circle to include not only family but also a wider world.

The toddler's sense that he can do it himself is more fully realized in the preschooler, who really *can* do many more things for himself. Dressing, going to the bathroom, feeding himself, riding tricycles or bicycles, and using scissors and paint with greater ease—all of these contribute to the young child's sense of pride and independence from you.

A preschooler's language and cognitive skills are much more developed than that of a toddler, which has both benefits and drawbacks. Now instead of simply saying "I'll be back at lunch time today," you can add, "That's in 3 hours," and it will mean something to him. Concrete markers of the passage of time are still helpful, though. If you must be away for several days, your child will be able to grasp approximately how long that is when you give him tangible clues. You might say, "I gave Grandma three pieces of bubble gum to give to you. You can chew one piece every day after lunch, and I'll be home on the day you have the last one." Children who are 4 or 5 can even begin to grasp the passage of days using a calendar. You can show your child how to mark off the days one by one until your return.

A preschooler is more likely to understand where you are going and when you will be back, and may be comforted by this. On the other hand, he is also a master of verbal manipulation. He will be able to come up with a dozen reasons why you really shouldn't go out on a particular night or why he doesn't want you to go away for a weekend even though his favorite aunt is coming to stay with him. Resist any temptation to negotiate the terms or conditions of your departure. Remember that you're the parent and the decision is yours to make. Be positive but firm about what's going to happen and when. In the long run, it will make goodbyes less stressful for everyone.

Once your child starts kindergarten or first grade, she will have one foot in her secure home base and another in the real world. Depending on her temperament and experience with goodbyes, she may happily trot off to be with her peers at school, playdates, and parties, or she may only reluctantly part company with you and her trusted caregivers.

As your child begins to feel more comfortable dealing with other adults, including teachers, the parents of friends, instructors, and relatives, he will no longer need you for the same things or in the same ways as he did when he was younger. Once he learns that he can comfortably turn to others to fulfill his needs, he will also become less hesitant about leaving you.

No matter what your child's age, however, changes such as a move to a new house, the birth of a sibling, or switching schools can throw her for a loop. Even minor events, such as the departure of visiting relatives or a return to routine after a week's sickness, may precipitate separation blues. And even if easy goodbyes characterized your partings in the past, you may find that she will protest or even act out if you try to leave when she's feeling that her universe is less than secure.

While new instances of separation may call for different responses on your part, the most important rule in the separation game is helping your child to understand that you will always be the secure home base she needs, whether she is riding the school bus for the first time, attending her first birthday party without you, going to sleep-away camp, or leaving for college. In the chapters that follow, some of the most common situations in a young child's life that require her to separate from you and other trusted caregivers are described, along with ways for you and your child to handle each one.

✿ TWO

The First Big Separation: Going Back to Work

A popular music video for young children features a song entitled, "My Mommy Comes Back." In the story that accompanies it, a mother in a business suit drops her daughter off with another mother who is minding several children in her home in a pleasant suburban neighborhood. The daughter hugs her mom goodbye and happily runs off to play. At the end of the day, when the little girl is busily coloring, she looks up to find her mother back from a day at work. There are kisses and hugs as the two happily head for home. But as all working moms know, leaving your child in the care of others from 9 to 5 isn't always smooth sailing.

Returning to work is probably the most difficult separation that faces working mothers. If you're a working mother, you've got plenty of company. Fifty-eight percent of moms with kids under the age of 6 work, most of them in full-time positions. There are a number of issues that can affect your comfort level and satisfaction with returning to work once your child is born. They include (1) how much gratification or stress your work brings you, (2) how well supported (emotionally and practically) you are by your husband and other important family members, (3) the quality of child care that you can find and afford, and (4) where your child is in terms of development and temperament. All of these topics are explored at length in this chapter.

There's an ongoing debate between psychologists about whether a mother's absence (because she works) affects her infant's ability to form a secure attachment (which makes healthy separations possible). One group maintains that infants who experience daily separations from their mothers are likely to interpret her absence as rejection, or they come to doubt their mother's availability and responsiveness (both of which are necessary to form a secure attachment).

Those who promote the "quality of mother" approach say that the fact that a mom works in and of itself is not the main factor in whether healthy attachments can be formed, but whether the dual role of mother and employee has a negative effect on a mother's ability to respond to her child. The working mother whose job and/or commute is so draining that her own emotional needs may interfere with her ability to be receptive to her child's needs in a timely way may make it difficult for the baby to form a secure attachment.

For most working mothers, however, the question of whether and when to return to work is one that is

dictated by company policy and financial circumstances. A 1995 study by the Families and Work Institute in New York City found that 55 percent of
employed women bring in half or more of their family's
income; 53 percent of those say they do not want to
give up any of their responsibilities at work or at home.
Still, angst comes with the territory. "Mothers are dis-
proportionately burdened with feelings of guilt about
leaving their children in someone else's care while
they go off to work," says Julia Robertson, M.D., child
psychiatrist and assistant professor at the University
of Louisville School of Medicine in Kentucky. "But if
you have invested years of training or working in your
field and working fulfills important needs of yours, you
will be operating from a position of mental equilibrium
and be able to give your children what they need,"
she adds.

That doesn't mean, however, that it will always be
easy to say goodbye as you run off to work. But if you
and your child were never anxious or sad over these
daily partings, something would be wrong. "You don't
want your child to be indifferent about separation,"
says Dr. Martha Cox. "Separations are both upsetting
and endurable where the bond between parent and
child is strong. In a good situation, the child develops
a sense of trust that her mother will always come
back," she says.

If you keep your guilt in check and work at achiev-
ing goodbyes that are both ritualistic and consistent,
leaving your child home in the care of a sitter or dropping her off at daycare can go smoothly and allow
both of you a chance to enjoy the social and growth
experiences you have when you are apart.

Do You Enjoy Your Work?

Whether you feel strongly stressed and anxious depends a lot on your satisfaction with your role as a working mother. Research indicates that mothers who are employed because they want to be and mothers who are home because they want to be are more likely to have securely attached children than are mothers who are in either role only because they feel they must be, according to Marsha Weinraub, Ph.D., professor of psychology at Philadelphia's Temple University. "The mother who resents being at home, who feels a bit martyred by her role in having to constantly meet the demands of a baby, is not going to be responsive. On the other hand, the mother who cannot wait to be with her child once she gets home from work is going to be able to be a better parent," says Dr. Weinraub.

Three months after Michelle Weber's son James was born, she went back to work. Even though both she and her husband worked, Michelle (not her real name) had the more secure job and was on the faster track because she had an MBA; her husband had a Ph.D. in English literature. Besides that, Michelle loved her work. But it took Michelle 9 months and three family daycare providers to find the right situation, one that James stayed with until he went to kindergarten.

Now, 8-year-old James is in the second grade, and Michelle has the benefit of hindsight. "James was the classic difficult child; he had such difficulties with transitions that we went to see a psychologist about it when he was between 1 and 2 years old. She told us there was nothing wrong with him, that he simply had the temperament of a difficult child. Goodbyes continued to be tough on him until he was about 4 years old," says Michelle.

Eight-year-old James is doing well in school, is a good athlete, and has good friends. "I don't know if he would feel more secure now if I'd been able to stay at home," admits Michelle, "but I know that I'm a happier person because I am working."

"The key to any child's happiness is whether his or her parents are happy and their needs are being met," says Dr. Robertson. "If their jobs are crucial factors in fulfilling emotional and financial needs, they are going to have the mental equilibrium they need to meet their child's needs," she says. Like Michelle, if you get more of a reward than just a paycheck from working, you will probably find that it's worthwhile to navigate through the inevitable ups and downs you're likely to go through finding and keeping the right child care. If, on the other hand, your job or work situation is unsatisfying and you have doubts about whether your child is being properly cared for, you may be a candidate for staying at home.

From Full-time Mom to Working Mom

Leaving your baby or child in the care of others isn't always a gut-wrenching decision; mothers who have established careers and enjoyed their work before making the decision to be at home with their child sometimes discover that they're ready to go back to work earlier than they had planned to.

Susan Gordon returned to work 3 months after the birth of her daughter, Mia. "It was hard leaving her all day, and I often cried on the way to work," remembers

Susan. Her separation anxiety peaked when Mia was about 11 months. "I felt that she wanted to be with me, and I wanted to be with her. She just had a whole different set of needs that were not met so perfectly by a caregiver," says Susan, who quit her job not long thereafter. She worked as a free-lance writer and editor and had a sitter come in part time.

Eventually, however, she discovered she missed the atmosphere and perks that came with being a magazine editor. When the right job offer came along 2 years later (Mia was then 3), Susan went back to work, although she had just found out that she was pregnant. "My husband and I found a terrific daycare center, and Mia really enjoyed being with other children all day. And I found out that it was much easier to leave Lilly 6 weeks after her birth than it was Mia," says Susan. "That's because I had learned that they were okay without me, so long as the care they were getting was first rate. And I feel like I'm a better parent because I am stimulated by my work and treasure the time that I have with my daughters at night and on weekends."

The Importance of Support

Another factor that contributes to how much stress you're feeling with your return to work is how much backup—emotional and practical—your spouse gives. "The amount of support a working mother gets from her spouse has a direct impact on how overloaded or satisfied she feels about her dual roles as parent and employee," says Dr. Cox.

Michelle Weber knows that firsthand. Up until the

time her children were in second grade and kindergarten, her job required far more hours and business travel than her husband's job did. He was the one who had to be sure to pick the children up from daycare and later, to relieve the sitter who took the children home from school. "If Les hadn't been the kind of guy who was willing to pitch in and help out, I could never have worked for the demanding, start-up companies I did," says Michelle.

Beyond the fact that a husband's support allows a working mother to have a demanding job that she finds challenging and rewarding, it's a plus for children, too. "A father's participation in caregiving can make a big difference in creating a strong and positive attachment to him as well as to their mother," says Dr. Stana Paulauskas. "And the more positive attachments children have to adults, the more secure they are as individuals and better able they are to function with adults outside their immediate family," she says.

Ingredients for Healthy Goodbyes

It's up to you as the parent to structure a successful goodbye. "You have to send the message to your child that you are in charge, that you trust the situation you are putting your child in, and that it's okay for the two of you to be apart for a while," says Carol Seefeldt, Ph.D., professor at the Institute for Child Study at the University of Maryland in College Park. When you let your child know that you expect him to be able to handle saying goodbye, it helps your child to build confidence and competence.

Parents who have successfully negotiated goodbyes

that work say that being consistent and sticking to a routine is critical. "I am not a particularly structured person, but I learned the hard way that my daughter Amy was much better able to say goodbye when events leading up to us separating were predictable," says Leigh Ann Schevchik. When Leigh Ann drops 3½-year-old Amy off at her Montessori school, she leaves her at the door to the classroom, asks if there is anything she wants to say before they say goodbye, then gives her a hug and a kiss, and is gone. "If I try to kiss her before I asked if she has anything to say, she'll correct me and tell me which step I've missed," says Leigh Ann.

What your routine is matters much less than having a script that, like an actor or actress, you faithfully perform each day. If your child leaves the house with you and the goodbye takes place at a daycare facility or preschool, your routine should start with the time at which you rouse your child. Be consistent in how you get him or her out of bed and accomplish the getting-ready tasks of eating breakfast, using the bathroom, and getting dressed.

Some parents find that using a kitchen timer helps their children keep track of what they need to do to accomplish a particular part of the getting-ready routine. Others award stickers or points (useful for 4- and 5-year olds) for getting-ready tasks that are successfully completed. The stickers may be rewards in and of themselves, or points may count toward an end-of-the-week reward.

Leaving the house can present its own set of delays, particularly for the child who wants to postpone separating from you, so the more pat you have that aspect

of the routine down, the better. A few general rules of
thumb here:

- Don't threaten to leave your child home alone if he
  won't walk out the front door with you.
- Limit your use of bribes (whether it's a lunch-box
  treat or promised toy) to speed up the exit process,
  or you'll soon discover that bribes become an expectation.
- Be firm and keep your voice under control even if
  your child is moving like a tortoise (showing how
  upset you are is likely to escalate foot dragging into
  a full-blown standoff).
- Don't ever expect your child to respond more quickly
  if you focus on your needs ("You're going to make
  me late for work") rather than his. You're far more
  likely to get cooperation if you empathize but stress
  your child's competence by saying, "Look, I know
  it's hard to get going this early, but you're a big boy,
  and it makes me proud of you when you're ready
  on time."
- Use a distraction maneuver. If you suspect that your
  child is trying to avoid walking out the door, get her
  mind off the imminent goodbye by talking about
  something you know will interest her. It might be
  picking out a special toy to take with her for sharing
  time, or a discussion about an upcoming family outing or what she'd like the two of you to do when
  you're back home together later in the day. Walk (out
  the door) as you talk.
- If none of these tactics work, you may have to pick
  your child up and carry her out. That can be physically and mentally exhausting, but try to keep your

cool, even if your child is kicking or hitting you. Saying goodbye will be easier for both of you if you haven't lost it and yelled at or spanked her.

Once you've arrived at the daycare center, the home of your family daycare provider, or a school, stick to your drop-off routine. "Rituals are extremely important to children," says Dr. Robertson. "Think of them as steps that help your child make a transition." Put your child's lunch in her cubby, help her off with her coat, and get her involved in an activity—or leave that up to the person in charge. Just be consistent. If you linger at the block table one day because you have the time or because you're feeling guilty because you got home from work late the night before and didn't have enough play time with your child, you're not doing your child a favor by modifying the routine. When she's having a tough day, she won't be able to understand why you cannot accommodate her. So tell her you love her or that you will be thinking of her; give her a hug, kiss, or high-five; and let her know when she will see you again.

COMFORT WITH CHILD CARE

How comfortable you feel with the quality of care your child is receiving is another major factor in your stress level. Research conducted at the Yale University Bush Center in Child Development and Social Policy in New Haven, Connecticut, indicates that the more satisfied mothers are that their children are being well cared for in their absence, the less anxious they feel.

When I began to try to visualize the sort of person

I wanted to care for my son, I imagined a combination of Mary Poppins, Mrs. Doubtfire, and my favorite grandmother. Then I began to worry that if I found her, he might fall in love with her! I discovered I wasn't the only mother who felt that way. After basic care and safety issues, the number-one concern of mothers who rely on someone else to provide child care for their infants is that the baby will get confused about who her primary caregiver is or, worse yet, that she will love her more than she loves you.

While this is a common concern, it is an unfounded fear. The opportunities for attachment are very different for moms than they are for caregivers. You are with your child much more often, and for much more important events: the morning smiles from the crib and sleepy 2 A.M. feedings, running errands together on a Saturday, even a quiet snuggle when your child has a cold or ear infection. No matter how fond your child is of his caregiver, he will prefer Mom or Dad. Even very young children are able to tell the difference between parents and important others.

No matter which type of care you choose, it's critical to get the highest-quality care you can afford. Studies show that child-care centers in states with stricter regulations were of a higher quality than those in states with loose or nonexistent licensing requirements. While licensing alone doesn't guarantee quality, it is more likely to mean that a center has features that are important to good outcomes: a good child/staff ratio; small group sizes; clean, safe facilities and equipment; and caregivers who have received early-childhood education.

Pros and Cons of Child-Care Options

AN IN-HOME NANNY OR LIVE-OUT SITTER

Pros:

* Your child gets plenty of one-on-one attention.
* You control the cleanliness and safety of the environment.
* You choose the individual who cares for your child.
* You can decide how you want the caregiver and your child to spend their time.
* You do not have to transport your child.

Cons:

* Good caregivers command good salaries or hourly pay.
* You have the responsibility of tax, insurance, and workers compensation matters when the caregiver is 18 or older and earns more than $1,000 a year.
* You may have to make backup arrangements if a caregiver is ill, wants a day off, or suddenly finds another job.

FAMILY DAYCARE

Pros:

* The setting is homelike and presumably safe and clean.
* Costs are more reasonable than hiring your own sitter because they are shared.
* Your child gets to play with other children.

Cons:

* While providers may be required to be licensed, care is not regulated, and the provider may lack formal training in child development.
* Your child must share the attention of the care provider with other children, which can be a plus or minus, depending on child's age.
* You may have to make backup arrangements if the care provider is ill or unable to provide care on a given day.
* Your child will be exposed to colds and other childhood illnesses.
* You will have to transport your child to the provider's home.

CENTER-BASED CARE

Pros:

* Staff at high-quality centers are likely to have training or education in child development.
* Care is still available when a staff member is sick or takes a day off.
* Cost is desirable because it's shared by many parents.
* Good equipment and facilities are available at high-quality centers.
* Your child gets to play with other children.

Cons:

* You will not usually not be able to choose your child's individual care providers.
* At less well run facilities, the ratio of care providers to infants or children may be larger than desirable (one care provider per three infants is recommended).

- Turnover among staff is high (often because wages are low).
- Your child will be exposed to colds and other childhood illnesses.
- You will have to transport your child to the center.

Children in settings that meet these basic standards of quality perform better in many areas of child development, including social, cognitive, and vocabulary development. Says Dr. Jay Belsky, "Try to find a sensitive, responsible caregiver who will be around for a decent interval. The most important thing is the responsiveness of the caregiver; the least important thing is the setting."

A 1995 study by psychologists of hundreds of daycare centers in four states found that the care provided by most is so poor that it could interfere with children's intellectual and emotional development. Particularly at risk were infants and toddlers; almost 40 percent of the places they were cared for were rated poor. And only one in seven offered the kind of warm relationship that enables children to learn to trust adults and the intellectual stimulation that readies children for school. The centers that received the highest ratings were those with access to money provided by federal or state sources, universities, or employers who offered child care at the work site. The challenge for most parents is being able to discern when child care is of high quality and when it isn't. The same study found that 90 percent of the parents interviewed believed the care their child was receiving was good, while psychologists found most centers provided mediocre or poor care.

Your child's first year of life seems to be one of the most problem-fraught times for finding the right child-care situation. Part of the reason is that as a new mother or father, you may not be sure what the ideal situation is; another factor is that you may not know the right questions to ask of a care provider or how to evaluate differences in child-care centers. The checklists on the following pages can help you weigh the pros and cons of a daycare center or evaluate the qualifications of a caregiver. One indicator of quality is whether a daycare center is accredited by the National Association for the Education of Young Children.

Daycare Center Checklist

When you visit daycare centers you're considering placing your child in, be sure to observe and/or ask about the following things:

* What is the staff/child ratio?
* Do most staff members seem to genuinely enjoy their work?
* How does the staff discipline children who misbehave?
* Do the children seem happy and engaged?
* Do you feel comfortable with the way staff discipline children who are misbehaving?
* Are there enough supplies and equipment for all the children to use?

- Does the staff make an effort to involve all the children, particularly shy or unhappy ones, in activities?
- Do children seem to feel comfortable asking questions or going to the staff for help?
- Are infants held and talked to, or are they in high chairs, infant seats, or cribs?
- Do infants coo and babble, or are they quiet and listless?
- Are caregivers mostly talking to one other, or are they busy with the children?
- Is the setting either too quiet (children are subdued) or chaotic and too noisy?
- Is there variety in the types of materials available (for music, small- and large-motor skill development, art, cognitive skill development)?
- Are there any visible health or safety hazards?

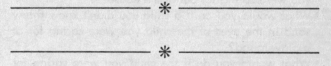

What to Ask a Prospective Caregiver

- What kind of experience have you had working with children?
- How long and how often did you do it?
- How old were the children you cared for?
- What did you like most and least about taking care of children?
- Are you currently working?
- Why do you want to leave your current situation (if working)?
- How long have you been looking for a job (if not working)?

* Why are you interested in this job?
* How many years have you been driving?
* Do you have a valid U.S. driver's license?
* Have you ever received a ticket or been involved in a traffic accident?
* Do you own your own car?
* Can you produce documentation about your car insurance and coverages?
* Are you a smoker? If so, how much do you smoke a day? How long a period can you go without having a cigarette?
* What kinds of things do you like to do with children who are my child's age?
* What would you do if a child you were caring for begin choking on his food?
* What would you do if you locked yourself and the child you were caring for out of the house?
* What would you do if a child you didn't know threw sand in the eyes of the child you were caring for at a playground?
* What would you do if the child you were caring for fell down and cut open her chin?
* How would you handle a child who was having a temper tantrum?

When interviewing a candidate who has applied to come to the United States under an au pair program approved by the federal government:

* Have you ever lived away from home before? under what circumstances, and for how long?
* Do you have any hesitations about being away from home for 1 year?
* Are you romantically involved with anyone at the current time? How does he/she feel about your going

away? (Missing that person can be a greater factor than homesickness and may result in a truncated stay.)

* How do you like to spend your free time?
* What are you most likely to be doing on a weekend night?
* Are you the kind of person who needs a lot of privacy/ time alone?
* Are you the kind of person who feels happier amusing yourself with something at home or going out (if you have free time)?
* How would you describe the usual condition of your room or apartment?
* What kind of exercise/physical activity do you like best?
* Are you the kind of person who is chipper or slow to wake up in the morning?
* Do you drink alcoholic beverages when you are out with your friends for the evening? How much do you drink?

———————— ✳ ————————

———————— ✳ ————————

Questions to Ask of References

If you're considering hiring a sitter to care for your child in your home or using a family daycare provider, be sure to contact references to make sure that the candidate you're considering hiring is honest, experienced, and has no skeletons in the closet. Parents for whom the caregiver has worked before can best answer the following questions:

- How would you describe your child's relationship with _____?
- Has she/he had experience caring for infants? toddlers? preschoolers?
- What kinds of things does she/he do with them?
- Does she/he need a lot of direction, or can you rely on her/him to take initiative?
- Were you unable to use her/his services for any period of time because she/he was ill?
- Would you describe her/him as someone with a lot of common sense and good judgment?
- How affectionate is she/he with children?
- Would you trust her/him to do the right thing in an emergency situation?
- What one or two things about her/him do you wish were a little different?
- Why did you stop using her/him for child care?

MONITORING YOUR CHILD-CARE CHOICE

Once you have hired a sitter or your child has started daycare, be sure to keep yourself informed about what happens every day in your child's new world. Set aside 10 or 15 minutes at the beginning and end of every day to touch base with your caregiver—after all, you and she are now partners in your child's care. Before you leave in the morning, make sure she knows about things that might affect your child's day, whether it's the fact that your child will probably need more nap time because teething pain interrupted her night sleep schedule, or that she's feeling sad because Grandma and Grandpa had to delay their visit. At the end of the day, the information exchange should go the other way, as your caregiver fills you in on your child's day. If he doesn't volunteer the kind of information you want to know, ask.

Finally, show up a few minutes early from time to time to see what's going on at home when you are not expected or to observe your child in a daycare setting (preferably without your child's catching sight of you). If you are disturbed by anything you observe, talk to your sitter or the daycare provider about it. If you're on hand to witness your child crying or acting out in some way, don't jump to the conclusion that it's the fault of the care provider. If possible, watch to see how the caregiver handles the situation. If you cannot hide your presence and your child demands your attention or you feel that your interrupting what you're witnessing is a good idea, postpone asking questions until you and/or your child are calmer. When you do, find out what was happening before you walked in and what your sitter or the daycare provider had already done to calm or deal with your child. If the explanation does not satisfy you and corroborates earlier uneasiness you may have had about the level of care being provided, consider whether changing caregivers or centers is in your child's best interest.

WHAT TO EXPECT AT DIFFERENT DEVELOPMENTAL STAGES

Finding child care you can trust will make you and your child feel better about separations at any age, but some problems and solutions apply more to certain ages than to others. Here are some of the hallmarks of daycare separations for young children at different stages of development, and some tips for keeping the experience as positive as possible for you and your child.

AGE FLAG: INFANCY TO 6 MONTHS

Returning to work when your baby is 6 months or younger will definitely bother you more than it bothers her, provided, of course that you have found a good caregiving situation. Although you may weep all the way to work for a month, and feel your heart contract with love and longing every time you glance at your new little one's picture on your desk, separation is simply not a big issue for children until separation anxiety comes into the picture at about 7 to 9 months. "Very young children separate easily because they have not yet developed the concept that Mom is always there," says Dr. Kathy Nathan.

Martha Farrell Erickson, Ph.D., director of the University of Minnesota's Children, Youth, and Family Consortium in Minneapolis, elaborates: "The attachment between parent and child is not really well established until the second half of the first year of life. That's when being apart really becomes as important to the child as it is to the parent."

AGE FLAG: 7 TO 18 MONTHS

Annie Giles found an excellent family daycare provider to look after her son Ian 3 days a week while she was in graduate school. In the beginning, their routine seemed almost to be almost too easy to be true. "I cried a little when I left him at daycare during the first couple of weeks, but he was only 3 months old, and it didn't seem to bother him at all. He would just settle into the sitter's arms and sort of grin, and I was only gone a half-day each time, so I figured we had a great setup," Annie said.

One day when Ian was about 8 months old, the morning routine suddenly changed. "It was like someone had flipped a switch," Annie says, remembering. "I handed Ian to the sitter, kissed him goodbye, and turned to go—then, bang! Tears! Ian just howled. I took him back and cuddled and kissed him, but I had to get to a class, and he was still crying when I left. I was so convinced that I'd been doing him some kind of damage all along without realizing it that I shook halfway to school," she says.

Continuing a routine that you have already established can be hard enough when separation anxiety sets in, but starting a new one is likely to be more challenging. During the second half of your child's first year, and for a year or so thereafter, you will have to contend with your child's growing awareness of others and preference for you. Advances in his cognitive development at this stage mean that your child is more aware of your presence—and thus of your absence. So, if it's possible, be advised that returning to work on a part-time or full-time basis is likely to be more difficult for your child if you return to work at this stage in his development.

AGE FLAG: 18 MONTHS TO 3 YEARS

Child-development experts warn that a child who has had too little experience with separation up to this time may have a more difficult time acclimating to the major change in routine when a parent returns to work. "If you wait a long time to separate from your child or you haven't had many practice separations, it's more of a production for both parent and child," says Janine Wenzel Reed, Ph.D., a clinical psychologist in private practice in Los Altos, California.

Strategies for Smoothing the Transition

If you go back to work when your child is 2 or older, count on questions and maybe even protest. Still, if circumstances warrant your return to the work force, you can prepare your child for the change. "Don't feel obligated to justify what you're doing to your child," suggests Dr. Weinraub. Just state the facts: "It's time for Mommy to go back to work. It's something I need to do, and I will be helping Daddy earn money to buy things for all of us."

The fewer changes that occur, the easier the transition will be. If, for example, you can afford to have a sitter come into your home, your child will not have to get used to a new setting and learn to compete with other children for a care provider's attention or just to get along with them.

Focus on what your child, not you, will be doing during the day. Explain that a new sitter, whom she has already met (during an interview) or whom she will soon meet, will be coming to stay with her at home during the day. Tell her that she will still sleep in her own bed, watch the same videos, eat at the same time, and get to play with her friends.

If you plan to put her in a family or center daycare

situation, be sure to take her there for a visit if she has not seen it already. Remind her or explain in advance what it will be like in very simple terms: "There will be a lot of fun toys. You will get to meet new playmates. There is a very nice person named Miss Joanne who will take care of you and make you snacks."

Don't apologize or ask for your child's permission to return to work. "If you make that mistake, it will give your child an opportunity to protest," warns Dr. Weinraub.

Let your child know what the new daily routine will be—most important, the time of day you leave or drop her off and when you will return or pick her up. Be sure to sound positive and upbeat about the change. If your toddler detects any hesitation on your part, she is likely to feel ambiguous, too, and protest the transition more strenuously.

Keep in mind that toddlerhood is a time of great swings from budding self-reliance to complete dependency on you. The strong emotions these conflicts generate in toddlers seldom find their outlet in rational discussion. On some days, this may result in very real tears and tantrums, but on other days, you may get the sneaking feeling that you are being manipulated. Toddlers are splendid at coming up with a variety of creative ways to let you know that they want you to stay with them when it's time to say goodbye. The trick is to dealing with their increasingly sophisticated means of plucking at your heartstrings is to stand firm while acknowledging their feelings. Dr. Weinraub suggests saying "I know you're going to miss me, and I'm going to miss you. It's okay to feel sad, but crying won't help you feel better. What do you think you can do to help yourself feel better?"

The new fears that are so typical of normal toddlerhood (fear of the dark, big dogs, bugs, and more) can interfere with easy separations. Remember that your toddler's primal fear is that you will abandon or cease to love her. No matter how unlikely you know this possibility is, it's critical to reassure your child that as in the song "My Mommy Comes Back," you will always come home after work or pick her up from daycare. If you are going to be late, always let the caregiver know so she can tell your child that you are on your way. Otherwise, your arrival may be met with a storm of terrified tears. And never threaten to leave your balking or dawdling toddler behind if he doesn't behave himself or hurry up; in the end, this will only make him scared of letting you out of his sight.

Going Back When Your Child Is a Preschooler

AGE FLAG: 3 TO 5 YEARS

Going back to work when your child is verbal and has the capability of arguing with you about your decision can be challenging indeed. Many of the same rules that applied to toddlers about preparing your child for the change apply to preschoolers as well. Talk about the new routine weeks before you actually implement it. Be upbeat about it, and be sure to familiarize your child with the place or the person who will be taking your place while you are at work.

Even if your child seems willing to try out the new situation at first, he may decide that he doesn't like it nearly as much as he did being home with you. A verbal preschooler may try to persuade you with her own logic to abandon this new scheme. He may say, "I thought I'd like the daycare center, but the kids won't play with me, and my teacher is mean."

While it's a good idea to keep a running dialog with your child about what's going on at daycare (or at home with her sitter), it's not wise to let her view of the world make you feel guilty or even like rethinking whether you should be back at work. "You cannot go through the 'Should I quit?' debate with yourself every time your child has a bad day or you run into snags with your caregiving situation," cautions Dr. Julia Robertson. "If you have carefully made a decision about returning to work, then stick with it and try to work out ways of coping with each minicrisis as it arises," she suggests. If, for example, you have any doubts about the quality of your caregiving situation, by all means check them out, but deal with your manipulative child by being understanding but firm. You might say, "I'm sad that you aren't having a good time at daycare. I'll talk to Miss Logan about how you can join in the play. I bet she'll have some good ideas."

HELLO AGAIN CAN BE DIFFICULT, TOO

Don't be surprised if your baby, toddler, or preschooler is distant, irritable, or downright angry at you when you reunite at the end of your workday. Giving you the cold shoulder or acting out is often a child's way of letting you know that he's not happy that you left him in the first place and is typical of behavior during the first few weeks of your returning to work and leaving him in someone else's care. Some children even refuse to go to their parents when they arrive; they may busy themselves with an activity and ignore their parents. No matter how much you may have anticipated sweeping your child up in your arms and getting a big hug and kiss, don't let your disappointment interfere with your actions. Take cues from the daycare provider or sitter (who will help the child with your return if she's skilled). Or give your child a few minutes to say hello again. You might make some ordinary conversation, such as asking him what kind of structure he's building or compliment her on the beautiful pictures she's painting.

One of the hardest reactions to stomach is to have your baby cling to his caregiver when you walk in, arms open. This is all the evidence some parents need to convince them that their child loves the caregiver more. Not so, says Dr. Kathy Nathan. "Some children are fine until they see their parents again," she explains. "Then they feel safe enough to fall apart. You may get the impression that your child has been miserable all day. But that's usually not the case; the crying or clinging is an emotional reaction."

The best way to deal with a child who masks her delight at your return is to try to warm up to her slowly. Let her know that you know she's not feeling happy. Tell her you missed her and how happy you are to be with her again. If she's using wounding language such as "I hate you, Mom, for making me come here," remind her that you love her, and tell her that she makes you feel sad when she says that. You may, however, want to take advantage of the opportunity to ask her to name what it is she doesn't like about her day there. As tempting as it may be to criticize her behavior, however annoying it may be (kicking the seat in front of her all the way home), don't show your irritation unless she's doing something that will damage property or physically hurt herself or you. In the end, the chances are good her mood will change quickly if you make the effort to distract her and get her involved in something fun.

Switching gears from your working self to your parenting self isn't easy, but it's in your child's best interests if you can give her your undivided attention when you reunite. When Dr. Erickson's children were young and attended a family daycare center, she used to go home for an hour or so before picking them up. This gave her a chance to decompress, sort the mail, change clothes, and relax a little. "It was great! Then I was really ready to see my children and give them my full attention," she says. If you can't do this, put household concerns on the back burner until you and your child have had a chance to spend some time together. Delay dinner, leave the mail in the mailbox, and give your child your full attention and all the cuddling he wants for at least 20 or 30 minutes.

SICK KIDS, TOUGH GOODBYES

Few scenarios are more heart-wrenching for working parents than having to leave a sick child who is clingier and needier than usual or who may make a pathetic but persuasive argument that where you belong is with him, not at work. If the child is your first and you are not yet experienced at negotiating the ups and downs of childhood illness, you may indeed be tempted to stay home, even if you know your child is in the competent hands of a familiar sitter or a close relative. But giving in to your emotions or your child's pleas is not always a smart choice.

Lisa Nash worked from home several times when her oldest daughter Sarah was sick and under the age of 2. "I had an understanding boss and the kind of job that made it possible for me to work from home," says Lisa. "But I got calls all day long from my staff, and Sarah got a raw deal because I wasn't available to her all the time, and she couldn't understand that. By day's end, I was really strung out from trying to deal with problems at work via telephone and trying to meet Sarah's needs. I discovered that it was much better for both of us for me to go to work as usual on days she was sick because when I got home at night I had the energy to focus on her exclusively. Going through those experiences and learning what to expect with childhood illnesses made it easier for me to deal with going to work when my younger daughter Mary got sick, too," says Lisa.

Lisa developed several strategies to help her daughters get through sick days without her that you may find will work for you, too. She made tapes of herself singing their favorite songs and telling stories. Lisa also got out family photo albums for Sarah to look at with her sitter. And she asked close family members to call and talk to her daughters when the girls were sick. Lisa also told them that she would take their phone calls at her office, which was an exception to the normal rule of end-of-the-day and emergency calls only.

Kid emergencies can also provoke emotional reactions from you if you are called by your sitter or the daycare provider while you're at work. Lisa got a panicky call one morning at work from her trusted sitter, who told her that 2-year-old Mary had mistaken 25 fluoride pills for candy and eaten them all. Lisa instructed her to call their pediatrician, follow his instructions, and call her back within 20 minutes. "I figured that he would either tell my sitter to give Mary syrup of ipecac (which causes regurgitation) or tell her to go to the emergency room, and I couldn't get home quickly enough to help with either of those solutions," says Lisa. She waited for 19 minutes, car keys in hand; then, unable to handle the suspense a moment longer, called home. The syrup of ipecac had worked, and the crisis was over. "In an emergency, I can really focus on how to solve the problem, but once I knew things were okay, I had to leave the office and take a walk because I was so drained emotionally," says Lisa.

How you react to an emergency helps your child know how to react, too. If, like Lisa, you can remain calm and in control (in talking to your child over the phone from your office, for example), your child will probably not think of what's happened as a big deal. If, on the other hand, you rush home in the middle of the day and are emotionally distraught about what's happened, she's likely to model that behavior.

WHEN SEPARATION PROBLEMS PERSIST

The child who is anxious about having his parents leave or being left in a new situation with adults he doesn't know well is behaving normally. So is the child who registers a protest, whether it's tears, clinging, or saying "Don't go." Preschoolers for whom separation is tough often act out their sadness or anger by refusing to talk or say more than a few words to their daycare providers and the other children, although they may talk nonstop at home. What's not normal is when these behaviors don't diminish in intensity and duration within a reasonable period of time. Most experts say that the majority of children adjust within 1 or 2 weeks' time to a new daily schedule that involves saying goodbye to one or both parents.

If your child continues to protest leaving you by refusing to get dressed or cooperate in activities leading up to the departure, throwing a tantrum, or displaying other inappropriate behavior when you leave, or excessively monitoring your comings and goings around the house, it's a good idea to try to figure out if these behaviors may be symptomatic of other stress he is experiencing.

Your child may also show stress through regressive behaviors, including refusing to get dressed without assistance, crawling into your lap at every opportunity, reverting to baby talk, following you from room to room, or demanding help with tasks she's capable of doing by herself. "If a regressive behavior goes on for more than a few days, you should look into what's going on," says Dr. Carol Seefeldt. "What children most fear is being deserted, and if, for example, they overhear a parental squabble, they may not only jump to the conclusion that they somehow caused it but worry that if Mommy and Daddy fight, they might get divorced, and then who will take care of them?" she says.

If you cannot put your finger on what's going on and the inappropriate behavior continues, you might benefit from professional advice. "Any disturbing or regressive behavior that is persistent and that is causing you or your child distress is worth exploring with a professional," says Dr. Robertson. Children cannot always express what's worrying them, and professionals are trained to know how to ask questions that elicit information that may be helpful in mediating the behavior.

Where to Find Help

There are several ways to track down good leads on professionals who can help you solve a temporary goodbye or stress-related crisis. "The key is to find someone who can take an objective look at the situation, identify what's going on, and suggest steps you can take to solve the problem," says Dr. Robertson.

The professional whose help you're seeking could be a child psychologist or psychiatrist or a social worker, according to Dr. Robertson. The most important criterion is that the person have training and experience working with children who are your child's age. Word-of-mouth recommendations from parents who have had a positive experience with a particular professional are the best leads. The director of your child's school or daycare facility may be able to provide the names of counseling facilities, if not the names of individual counselors. If you need additional leads, look in your phone book for a local chapter of the American Psychiatric Association, the American Psychological Association, or the National Association of Social Workers. These organizations often provide referrals, although they do not usually have the resources to match you with just the right person. Some phone books also list community-service organizations in the color-coded sections of the phone book. Look under the "Counseling" heading. Be sure to interview professionals to whom you are referred about their experience, clientele, and the types of problems with children and parents that they typically treat before you decide to work with that person.

WHEN A CRISIS STRIKES

Few events are more traumatic for parents than having something bad happen to their child while she is being cared for by someone else. You are likely to feel angry, helpless, and guilty. "You have to remember that accidents and children hurting your child may just as easily happen when you're around as when you're not," says Dr. Robertson. "What's important is for [you] to send the right message to your child: that even though bad things happen, you can get on with your lives," she adds. That's what Lisa Forchay (not her real name) did when her 21-month-old daughter, Whitney, was attacked by a 120-pound dog.

"When my daughter Whitney was born, I was halfway through my MBA and working at a job I really liked and didn't want to be mommy-tracked," says Lisa. "But it was critical to me to find a nurturing and stimulating daycare situation for my child." She found the perfect situation: a friend who became Whitney's godmother and was at home with her own young children.

"I never thought twice about whether Whitney was safe; I knew that my friend was trustworthy," says

Lisa. But one day the caregiver's Akita, who was usually not indoors, was allowed into the house, separated from the children by only a kid gate. When Whitney went into the gated area to hug him, the Akita bit her on her face and ear. The wounds required more than 30 stitches, nine local injections of anesthesia, and an hour of plastic surgery. "I couldn't go back to work for 10 days after it happened," remembers Lisa. "My husband and I also decided not to change our daycare situation. The caregiver and her family loved Whitney, they had the dog destroyed, and they were grieving about what happened as much as we were. But did I ever get flack from friends and colleagues who couldn't believe that I wasn't changing caregivers and suing my friend. They made me feel like a bad mom, but I tried to think of Whitney's needs first, and I decided that changing the only caregiver she'd known would be a big mistake."

That response was the right one, says Dr. Robertson. "A disruption in the caregiving situation and a child's attachment to important people in her life could have been a second trauma. It's very important for parents to model appropriate behavior so that the child can get through the trauma, too."

GUILT AND GOODBYES: A FINAL WORD

Being a working mom (or parent) may be one of the toughest regular separations you have to endure during your child's early years. But if you have made the decision to do it, you have nothing to gain and much to lose by letting your anxiety about your child's well-being consume part of your worry quotient every day, provided that you are confident about the quality of care your child is receiving. "Being a working mother provides tremendous opportunity for guilt and misery," says Michelle Weber, who did not interrupt her career once her children were born. "But you have to keep asking yourself whether you are making the best trade-offs you can at any point in time so that your children are happy and well cared for. I believe that if you are a loving parent, your children will know that."

In fact, guilt can actually interfere with your ability to help your child make smooth transitions to and from daycare or a school situation. "Guilt disables your coping skills," says Dr. Robertson. "You have to be outwardly focused on your child and his or her emotional state. If you are fighting your own strong, painful emotions about leaving your child to go to work, you will not have the energy to focus on what your child needs, and you are likely to be inconsistent in your behavior toward your child as you say goodbye," she adds.

What good goodbyes are all about is limit setting, rituals, regularity—strict rules about the kinds of behavior you will and will not tolerate and planned steps that you help your child take each day to help her achieve a sense of competence and independence that will serve both your needs.

Guidelines for Work-at-Home Parents

If you work at home and have a sitter come in to tend to your little one's needs, take these suggestions to heart:

- Don't make the mistake of thinking you can get work done at home without having someone care for your child. It may work for a while with a newborn, but you'll soon discover that your work will revolve around your child. If you have deadlines to meet or a boss to please, this arrangement will not work.

- Explain and, when necessary, reinforce the idea that even though you are at home, you are only available to your child at certain times. Close your office door (lock it if necessary) and hang a Do Not Disturb sign on it that you teach your child to recognize. Make your visitations to your child at predictable times (lunch, after his nap, when he returns from nursery school) so that he knows when to expect to see you.

- With an infant, popping in and out as your time and desire allows is fine. But think about making your appearances more regular once she's 6 to 8 months old and separation anxiety sets in.

- Instead of inviting your child into your workspace (where he will, at some stage, get into things you don't want to share), go to his space.

- Make sure your sitter understands her role in distracting your child from coming to see you. If you're consistent and you communicate when interruptions are welcome or not, your relationship will work better, and the possibility of unwanted intrusions will be kept to a minimum.

- Avoid bending the rules when "in-house" goodbyes become difficult. If your child learns he can make you come to him by crying, throwing a tantrum, or manipulating his sitter, you'll have much bigger goodbye problems to solve.
- Even if the location of your office allows you to slip out unnoticed by your child and her caregiver, it's far better to say goodbye so that your child learns that when you say goodbye, you will return again.

🌀 THREE

"Dates" with Mates and Friends

No strict father, overprotective big brother, or teasing little sister ever interfered with the course of true love—or at least dinner and a movie on Saturday night—the way your tiny, cooing darling or adorable toddler can. If you left it up to your child, you would not be allowed to go on dates with your mate or catch an occasional night out with a good friend.

The protest you encounter may make you wonder if it's worth the trouble. Why not just order in a pizza, put the kids to bed early, and pop in a rented video? For many parents, finding a sitter and going out for fun is harder than leaving their child when it's time to go to work. Work, after all, is a non-negotiable necessity; going out at night with one's partner (or worse yet, one's friends!) is a self-indulgent option, right? Wrong.

"Martyrs don't make great parents," says Dr. Mar-

tha Farrell Erickson. "It is important for parents to
get some respite and to have a life beyond parenting.
It's really important for parents to feel rested and re-
freshed. Then they can be more emotionally available
when they are with their child."

Meeting the needs of children on a constant basis is
the most demanding job in the world, one from which
you need breaks. Enjoying a meal without having to
cut someone else's meat and being able to wear a
blouse with no strained peaches on the sleeves may
not be an inalienable right, but it can help you to be a
happier—and thus better—parent. It is not only possible but desirable to acknowledge and work on meeting
your own needs without compromising your child's
well-being.

Taking a break from parenting isn't the only good
reason to go out; spouses need time together to nurture their relationship. "It's really critical for parents
to step out of their dad and mom roles and into their
husband and wife roles," says Dr. Janine Wenzel Reed.
"It's a big mistake to neglect your couple relationship,
because the stability of the family unit rests on the
couple's relationship." Dr. Reed, who is also the
mother of two, acknowledges that it is tempting to put
off plans if your child screams and protests at the very
mention of staying with a sitter. But it's also a bad
idea: "The problem is that if you don't follow through
with your plans to go out, it gets more difficult because
the child has learned that he can manipulate you to
stay if he protests long and hard enough," she adds.

Spending time away from your child benefits him,
too. "It's important to teach a child that others can
care for him, too, and that Mom and Dad will come

back," says Barbara Talent, Ph.D., clinical psychologist at the Child Development Center at St. John's Mercy Hospital in St. Louis, Missouri.

GET OUT WHILE THE GETTING IS GOOD

AGE FLAG: NEWBORN TO 6 MONTHS

During the first 6 to 8 months of your baby's life, going out without baby is a bit like a kind of grace period during which you can get out without much protest from your child. She may cry briefly or gaze for a few moments at the door through which you have departed, but she will quickly be distracted by whatever toys and games her caregiver has to offer.

So establish a routine of time out alone with your spouse early on, even though you may feel reluctant to leave your baby with a caregiver. Take the time to find a person you can trust, then set up a pattern of getting out on a regular basis, even if it's only once a week with your husband or an afternoon with a friend. Dr. Reed recommends that you start your dating life as parents by the time your child is 3 or 4 months old.

Even if you are breast-feeding, you can still get away for short times, or express milk for the sitter to give your child if you are out for more than 2 or 3 hours. The bonus to starting this pattern early in your baby's life is that even after separation anxiety becomes a factor, he will have become accustomed to both your departures (helping him to develop a sense of trust that you will return) and to his caregivers. Both will make your going out more tolerable to your child than trying to start at a later point.

Although you may be tempted to leave your little

one once you have bedded her down for the evening, don't be lulled into the "she won't even know I'm gone" mindset. Even a very young infant will be surprised if she wakes up 1 or 2 hours into sleep and has her diaper changed or feeding offered by someone she does not recognize. If your baby will be going to bed before you go out, have the caregiver come early and spend some time cuddling him while you are still there. Then you can put him to bed as usual, and go out feeling more comfortable knowing your child won't be alarmed if you are not there when he awakens.

Whether you're eager to share a glass of wine and a gourmet meal with your spouse or less than eager to leave the warm little form cocooned in the bassinet, don't be surprised if your thoughts and conversation return to baby. When David and Nancy Howell went out for the first time after the birth of their first child, they were so starved for nonbaby conversation that they decided they wouldn't even talk about their new son. Having dinner in a bistro with butcher paper covers on the tables, they used the crayons on the table to play a game of "hangman" while they waited for their dinner. The first word David chose? The name of their new son.

AGE FLAG: 6 TO 18 MONTHS

After our first child was born, my husband and I delayed going out on a date until he was 4 months old. Despite my concerns about his reaction, the only tears shed as my husband and I trouped off to dinner were mine. We went out a few weeks later, then again, then again. Having some time to ourselves seemed like a piece of cake. Then one night as we breezed out the door, waving goodbye to our now 7-month-old son, came The Meltdown. He cried, he wailed, he reached for me with both arms and a look of what I interpreted as utter betrayal.

By 7 or 8 months of age (and in some babies, as early as 6 months) your baby will prefer Mom and Dad above all others and will use the powers at her disposal to keep you nearby. And for such a tiny creature, the tool she has for preventing separations—lung power—may not persuade you to stay, but it sure can make you feel guilty about leaving. Many a conversation en route to a restaurant or movie theater has been spent on what's going on "back at the ranch" instead of the date chatter that is what makes getting away so much fun.

Relax—the crisis provoked by your departure is a fleeting one. If you handle such outings carefully, your child not only will be fine, but will develop a stronger sense of trust in you and your certain return. Successful time away from your child involves two things—the way you say goodbye and the quality of the care your child receives when you are gone. Even a baby who cannot yet speak picks up on the messages of comfort and calm conveyed by your tone of voice and in your body language.

The most important difference between minding the baby in the first half-year of life and the second half and beyond is that the older child is aware of—and may be wary of—the difference between parents and strangers. Even his accustomed sitter may get a few apprehensive looks from your newly vigilant 8-month-old if he hasn't seen her in a few weeks. And the intro-

duction of a new sitter may provoke cries and clingi-
ness. This is especially likely to be so if your child is
sensitive to changes in his routine.

Further complicating this already complex situation
is your baby's new mobility. The attainment of developmental milestones such as crawling and walking are
typically associated with temporary increases in clingi-
ness. It is as if your child is saying "Just because I can
move away from you on my own doesn't mean that I
am ready for you to move away from me!" At this
time, even your going into the bathroom and shutting
the door may provoke cries and whimpers from your
young Mommy-seeking missile. Leaving the house
without him need not be a major trauma, but it will
require planning, finesse, and lots of extra reassurances on your part.

Just because your baby can't talk yet is no reason
not to prepare him for your leaving. Say, just as you
would to a slightly older child, "We're going to go out
for a few hours, sweetheart. Maryanne is here to look
after you. And when we get back, I'll come in and say
good night." Remember that body language and tone
of voice are just as important as the actual words you
use. If you are anxious, guilt-ridden, or tearful at this
short parting, your young one may pick up on your
nervousness and may become upset herself. If, on the
other hand, you are calm and soothing and your voice
is confident and warm, she will begin to get the message that such separations are no big deal.

PERFECTING DEPARTURES

AGE FLAG: 2 TO 3 YEARS

Once your baby becomes a toddler, the pleasures and pitfalls of getting away for a few hours double. Keeping up with newly mobile young children leaves even the most patient and energetic parent eager for a chance to recuperate. Some traits typical of toddlers will make short outings at this stage easier, while others will bring new challenges.

At about 24 months, your child will have a far greater capacity to express himself verbally. He will also have a more sophisticated grasp of what you tell him and a much greater awareness of—and desire to control—your comings and goings. Even as you use your verbal skills to soothe the separation blues for your child, he will be using his to try to prevent your departure, no matter how much he loves his sitter.

His sense of time, however, is still relatively undeveloped. Even if you said you would be home in 3 hours, it's hard for him to gauge that time, and he may begin to fret when you haven't come home after just an hour, feeling that whatever 3 hours means, it must surely be up by now.

The toddler's world is full of conflicting demands. He is driven by a greater sense of capability and independence but constrained by his inability to do certain things himself. A toddler's feelings, emotions, and desires run high. When he cannot express them with his developing verbal skills, they erupt through the only emotional overflow valve he has: a tantrum. Knowing how to handle a tantrum at the door can come in very handy. Here's what you can do:

- *Ignore it.* It's tough to do when your child is wailing like a banshee, but let her know that her behavior is not going to make you change your plans. Say, "I'm sorry that you feel this way, but I (or we) have to leave now. I'll come in and give you a good-night kiss when I get home." Give her a kiss or a hug. If that's not feasible under the circumstances, blow a kiss or wave goodbye. Go, and do not turn back.

- *Use a distraction maneuver.* This works best for heading off a looming tantrum than for stopping one in progress. If your child's lip starts to quiver as you head for the door, whisk out a favorite toy, point to the sitter, and say, "Did you show this jack-in-the-box to Mrs. Ramon? I'll bet she'd like to see how it works."

- *Enlist your sitter's help.* If your child's tantrum behavior is likely to include wrapping herself around you or following you out the door, tell your sitter in advance that she may have to act as a human strait jacket until you're gone and the door is safely closed. Let her know what works best for your child: putting him down if he's kicking or flailing, rubbing his back gently once the tantrum is subsiding, or putting on a video to attract his attention elsewhere.

No matter how upset your child is at the moment of your departure, it's highly likely that it won't be long before she's her old self. Most kids bounce back quickly from brief storms of tears.

AGE FLAG: 4 TO 5 YEARS

By the time your child is a preschooler, short-term separations that enable you to get out for an evening movie, an afternoon coffee with a friend, or a morning of volunteer work at your older child's school should be far easier. There may still be rough spots ahead, but the preschooler has several things going for her that make help her not only to take separations in stride, but even to look forward to them.

For one thing, your preschool child will have had ample opportunity to build on the good relationship you have developed with her. If you go out relatively often, she has had a chance to learn that you always come back when you say you will, and that people other than her parents can provide loving, safe, and fun care for her in your absence.

In addition, your preschool child is much further along in his linguistic and cognitive development than he was even a year ago. When you tell him "I'll be home in 2 hours," he has some grasp of what this means; if you strengthen the message by saying, "That's as long as it would take you to watch Lamb Chop four times," his understanding is that much more concrete.

The rewards of having a sitter are not lost on preschoolers, and this can make separations far easier for both of you. Children of this age have usually had enough experience with parents' nights out to realize that rules are a bit more relaxed when Mom and Dad aren't there, or they know that special treats or variations in routine are their reward for good conduct on date night.

Four-year-old David and his teenage sitter Katie, for instance, have been working on a drawing—an elaborate cityscape with skyscrapers and enticing-looking shops—for months. Whenever his parents go out, Katie makes a big bowl of popcorn, and she and David expand their city with markers and crayons. When David's parents tell him early in the week that they'll be going out to a movie on Friday night, his response is a triumphant "Yesss!" and his week is filled with excited questions: "How many more days till Katie comes? Is today the day that Katie's coming to draw with me?" By the time Friday night rolls around, he is so excited he goes with his mother to pick Katie up and has the markers and the popcorn popper out before his parents have even kissed him goodbye.

Of course, not all children look forward to an evening with a sitter the way David does, particularly if a sitter is someone who also cares for him all day long, or if their parents are going out after they have both worked all day. Preschoolers are skilled at constructing credible arguments for why you shouldn't go out or protesting that your date or time out with a friend is cutting into your time with her.

Listen to what she's saying, acknowledge her feelings, and, if possible, come up with a time-together solution. You might say, "You know, I hadn't thought of it that way. I have had dinner meetings every night this week, and I haven't been able to play with you. But neither have I had time to see your mom. Suppose we make this Saturday a family-only time? And can you come up with a couple of ideas on how you'd like to spend it with us?"

"WHY CAN'T I GO, TOO?"

AGE FLAG: 3 TO 5 YEARS

The right answer to "Why can't I go with you and Daddy?" depends on the age of the child doing the asking. For a 3-year-old, the best answer is a simple "Because we're going to a place that's just for grown-ups. You'll have a lot more fun here with Grandma."

The older child is going to want a better explanation, so you might add: "Because I need some time to play with Daddy (or Mommy) just like you need time to play with your friends."

Your child may complain bitterly if you are going out with friends who are the parents of his friends. Assure him that all of the children will be at home with sitters, just like him. If the event is at your friends' home, make sure he understands that your hosts' children will be going to bed just as he will.

When Lisa Forchay goes out with her friend, Sandra, once a week, her 5-year-old daughter Whitney starts to cry. "She doesn't mind if Sandra and I go out, but she's afraid that Sandra's daughter, who is her age and her friend, will be allowed to come and she won't, no matter how often I explain that it's just going to be the two of us," says Lisa. One tactic that has helped Whitney cope with her feelings is to write down how she feels and draw a picture that she leaves out for her mother. "It usually says, 'I'm sad. I miss you. Come back soon,'" says Lisa.

In general, it is a good idea to play down whatever you are going to be doing, lest it sound enviable to your child. When Peggy and Joe Tabacco's children were 4 and 5 years old and thought the idea of accompanying their parents to dinner sounded like a lot of fun, they were told that the dinnertime conversation would be about "wine, politics, and business," subjects the children disliked (but occasionally overheard at the supper table). The prospect of staying home with their sitter sounded preferable, particularly when they were promised popcorn, a new video, or some other kind of special treat if they behaved.

In fact, making sure that your child has something to look forward to can go a long way toward easing a goodbye. If you know from experience that your departure is likely to elicit a scene, use the special treat as an incentive for good goodbye behavior. But be realistic; you cannot expect a child for whom transitions are difficult to go from a clinging vine to a waving, beaming angel as you walk out. Again, tell him that it's all right for him to feel sad (even if it means a few tears), but be clear about what kind of behavior will win the reward: no clinging, no screaming, no misbehavior.

✳

Going Out Do's and Don'ts

Don't tell your child you need a break from him—even if it's true.

Do emphasize instead that you have some grown-up things to do or that you need to go out with your spouse or friends.

Don't say that your child has been so bad that you might not come back.

Do tell your child approximately when you'll be back, and give her some marker to help her understand the time (for example, "after you are in bed asleep," "after lunch time," or—if it's true—"in time to read you a story and tuck you in bed"). If you don't expect to be home until after her bedtime, tell her you will come in and kiss her (without waking her) as soon as you get home— then do it. (My 6-year-old still asks me, the morning after I've been out, "Did you come and kiss me even before you took off your coat?")

Don't make your night out sound so exciting that your child will be resentful or unhappy that he can't come.

Do stress what he and the sitter will be doing while you are gone.

Don't tell your child too far ahead of time that you are going out, especially if anticipating it is stressful for him.

Do take into account your child's temperament and developmental level in deciding when to let her know that you have plans. If she's the type who gets anxious well in advance, a notice of several hours is probably better for her than knowing for 1 or 2 days, for example. A verbal toddler who looks forward to a visit from the sitter can be told the morning of your evening date so that he doesn't drive you crazy asking if it's time for the sitter to arrive.

------------------------------ ✳ ------------------------------

WHY PARENT OUTINGS ARE HARD FOR SOME KIDS

Some children seem nonchalant by their parents' taking leave of them. They're happily at play when Mom and Dad come to plant a goodbye kiss on their heads. But such effortless goodbye scenes never seem to happen if a child is of a certain temperament—high emotional sensitivity and low adaptability to new situations or people.

Tom and Sue Schmidt were looking forward to going to Tom's twentieth high-school reunion. And 5½-year-old Alex and 4-year-old Eric were accustomed to having their parents go out on occasional dates. What would make their going out all evening easier (or so Tom and Sue thought) was that the family was at Tom's parents' home for a family reunion, and all eight of the boys' cousins were there. When Tom and Sue kissed the boys goodbye, however, Alex began to sob uncontrollably. "You and Mom are going out, but all my cousins' parents are staying? It's not fair," Alex choked out between tears. After 10 minutes of hugs and reassurances, Tom and Sue left. Although his aunts and uncles tried their best to distract him, Alex was inconsolable. His younger brother put his arm around him and said: "Alex, it'll be okay. They're coming back. They're only going to be gone a few hours." It took another 15 minutes before Alex could be cajoled into a ball game. He had fun that evening, but an undercurrent of sadness punctuated his play, and he cried again when one of his aunts put him down for the night because he missed his Mom and Dad.

"I can relate to how Alex feels because I was the same way when I was a kid," says Tom. "My parents went out to a dance most Saturday nights and I didn't like it even though I had a sister and two brothers to play with, the sitters were usually a lot of fun, and I knew my parents would come back."

When Alex's cousins departed before his own family did, Alex got teary-eyed, too. "Sue and I try to acknowledge Alex's feelings. I tell him, 'I understand how you feel; it's sad when you have such a good time playing with your cousins, and then everyone has to go home.' Then I try to talk about some of the things the cousins did together that were a lot of fun so that he can replace his sadness with good memories," says Tom.

A child's temperament is a good predictor of how upset she will get over these small separations and how easy it is for sitters to comfort them in your absence. If your child is a smooth sailer, altering his usual routine to include a night out for you will probably elicit only a minor protest that quickly diminishes—or perhaps no protest at all. If changes in routine make him anxious, however, he will probably do everything within his power to convince you that you should stay with him. It's important to recognize your child's feelings, but again, don't accommodate him to the point that you seldom go out.

How Often Should You Go Out?

Whether you go out once a week or once every 2 weeks is less important than going out on a regular basis. "A young child's sense of time is not well enough developed for her to notice what your schedule is," says Dr. Martha Farrell Erickson. The important thing about the timing and frequency of your dates is that they ought to occur frequently enough for them to become a routine and accepted part of your family life.

"If a child is not frequently left alone without one or the other parent being available, his or her reaction may be extreme," says Byron Egeland, Ph.D., professor of child development at the University of Minnesota. "If, however, the child's relationship with the parents is good, she will adjust to her parents' going out without her."

In addition to frequency, another predictor of how easily parents can go out is the comfort level the child has with the caregiver. The more familiar and liked that person is, the easier the goodbye will be, regardless of the child's temperament or age.

Peggy and Joe Tabacco found that the times when their children were most likely to react negatively to their going out on their weekly date night was when they had to use a new sitter who wasn't the same person who took care of the children during the day while they worked. "Most of the time, our kids took our going out in stride because they knew and liked their caregiver," says Peggy. "But every once in a while, that person wasn't available, and our then verbal kids would inevitably try to talk us out of going out or including them on our date. We tried to reassure them that they would have a good time with the new sitter, but we never let them persuade us to stay home."

Your Caregiver: A Major Factor in Date Success

Finding someone you can trust to take care of and entertain your child can be a tall order, particularly if you only plan to use her on an occasional basis. When you are new to an area or are a relative novice in the great sitter search, you may find yourself frustrated at tracking down good candidates.

Although word of mouth is one of the best ways to get leads on good sitters, parents who find reliable evening help are often reluctant to share their find with anyone else. One of my dearest friends has referred me to her pediatrician, her sons' barber, and her fresh-fish market, but I know her best sitter only by her first name; she won't tell me her last name or her phone number!

Sitters who have had experience caring for children who are your child's age, or who have siblings that age, are the best choice. One of the best ways to evaluate a prospective sitter is to observe her in action. When you interview her, make sure your child is awake. Watch how she interacts with your child and how he reacts to her. Use the information you've gathered both from talking with her and from checking her references, along with what your gut instinct tells you about her capability.

* * * * * * * ✳ * * * * * * *

Where to Find Part-Time and Occasional Sitters

Finding a reliable, trustworthy sitter requires ingenuity, perseverance, and some luck. Keep in mind that your chances of getting someone good increase if you can offer regular hours (twice a week from 6 to 9 P.M., for example) and pay slightly more than the going rate. Here are ways to locate candidates:

- Contact the office of the local high school and ask if you can post a notice or have a babysitting job announced.
- Call your local Red Cross chapter and ask if they offer a course in babysitting or CPR (cardiovascular pulmonary resuscitation) for children. Ask if they keep the names and numbers of those who successfully pass the course.
- Ask the caregivers at the nursery of a church or synagogue you attend whether they might be interested in doing part-time sitting.
- Check with community senior centers to find out if they keep a list of active retired people who babysit or if you can post a notice.
- Call the off-campus employment office (sometimes the career planning and placement office) of a nearby college or university to post the job. Or call Jobtrak ([800] 999-8725 or, in the 310 area code, 474-3377), a college job-listing service that posts job listings at colleges in 24 states (most extensively in California). A 2-week posting costs $12.50 per college.
- Talk to directors of nearby nursery schools to find out if any of their teachers might be interested in evening or weekend work. Preschool teachers usually earn modest salaries and may work less than full time, which makes them good candidates for sitting jobs (provided you're willing to match their hourly salaries).
- Ask friends who have au pairs whether they are receptive to letting their au pair do sitting for you when she's not "on duty." Many of these young women (who come primarily from Europe) are eager to make extra money beyond the stipend they receive (usually $125 per week). But be diplomatic and considerate in your demands on the au pair's time, or you may find that your friends quickly become resentful.
- Post a notice (with tear-off slips with your name and

phone number) at locations (shopping centers, libraries, bookstores) near your home. Just know that you will have to screen candidates more carefully since you're advertising to the "general public."

Be sure to talk to several references (preferably parents who have recently used or still use the services of the sitter you're considering) before you hire the person.

Before you leave a new sitter alone with your child, arrange for him to come an hour or so before you leave or have him do a try-out (of course, you should pay him in both instances). You might arrange to have him entertain your child while you do something around the house that requires uninterrupted time. Peek in every now and then without letting your child see you to observe how things are going.

Be sure to share your house rules and provide the names and numbers of people who you want the sitter to call if you are unreachable: a trusted neighbor, a close relative, or even your child's regular daytime caregiver. Write down or tell her things that will be useful to her: that your daughter prefers to drink her bottle while being rocked; that your son may put up a fuss when you leave but will quiet down easily if you pull out his favorite book; or that even though she's toilet-trained, she may need to be reminded that it's time to visit the bathroom.

Make it clear which rules your child must follow (teeth brushed before bed) and which ones can be stretched a little (a slightly later bedtime). And no matter what her age, let your sitter know that you do not want her to ask friends over (even after your child is in bed) or to make personal phone calls while she's on duty.

Only a Beep or Ring Away

Cellular phones and beepers may be the biggest contributors to peace of mind that parents out on the town can have. It's the best way of being accessible to home without interrupting a pleasant dinner or vying for a pay phone in a crowded theater. But be clear about when you want your sitter to contact you. You may want to make it on an emergency basis only, or you may want a new sitter to check in and let you know how things are going after 1 or 2 hours. If a goodbye has been horrendous, signaling the sitter to call you in a free minute to reassure you that calm has returned can make a difference in how much you enjoy the rest of the evening.

Of course, it's smart to go out of your way to keep a good sitter happy. Come home when you say you are going to (or call to let him know you're going to be a little late); pay him the going rate or more; give him plenty of advance notice about when you'll need him; make it a point to buy a food or two you know he likes; and, of course, tell him often what a good job he does. (Remembering his birthday doesn't hurt, either!)

Try a Babysitting Co-op

In some communities, babysitting cooperatives, or co-ops, are a great alternative to sitters for parents who want an occasional free night out and are willing to exchange their services. Here's how they work:

* Parents list their names, along with the ages of their children and the ages of the children they would be willing to care for; only other members of the co-op can have copies of the list.
* Arrangements can be informal or formal. For instance, members may start with 20 tickets, each redeemable for 30 minutes of child care from other members. Or members may simply call each other up and propose a date-night "swap."
* Members meet every month or so to talk about how well the co-op is working and to plan occasional group outings for everyone.

If you decide to join one, keep these things in mind:

* Don't get into a situation where you're contributing far more hours of care than you're using by taking advantage of your accumulated "credits."
* Try to select families whose children's ages will complement your own. They need not necessarily be the same age; an older child who is interested in toddlers is often a better playmate than another 2-year-old.
* Don't be afraid to talk to member parents you don't know well to find out if their discipline style, values, and involvement in play is compatible with your own.
* If you find one family with whom you happily exchange regular care, and your children weather sepa-

rations well under these circumstances, don't feel badly about not calling other co-op members.

• If more than one co-op family reports that your child has a hard time adjusting to being in their home or that he cried too much or acted out, think twice about whether a babysitting co-op is going to be right for you.

Dad's in Charge

Taking time to do some of the things you did solo in your free time before your children were a part of your life is important for your continued mental health as a parent and a spouse. Although no surveys have been done that measure which parent gets out more, anecdotal evidence suggests that dads are much more likely to continue playing in their softball league, golfing on Saturdays, or getting together with "the boys." And most don't feel guilty about it, either.

Denying yourself time to pursue coffee with friends (unless it's with a kid in tow), a game of tennis, or your monthly book club meetings is a mistake. "The mother whose husband has played a role in taking care of their child all along is going to have an easier time with goodbyes, and so is the child," says Dr. Martha Cox. "When there are two secure attachments in a child's life, he is twice blessed and buffered," she adds.

Barbara and Jack Watson (not their real names) learned that reality the hard way. "I was a full-time stay-at-home mom, and my husband Jack didn't spend that much time with our two girls when they were babies and toddlers," says Barbara. "When I began to get active in Junior League and started going to evening meetings when my girls were 2 and 4, they protested loud and clear." As soon as Barbara headed for the door, the girls yelled, "Mommy, Mommy, don't go out; don't leave us," and yanked on her clothes. Jack had to restrain the 2-year-old so that Barbara could walk out the door. "As I watched them pounding on the windows and screaming, and I saw what a hard time my husband had controlling them, I felt guilty and wondered whether I should just bag the meetings," remembers Barbara. "But I decided the three of them should learn how to enjoy an evening together, and I should be able to do something I really wanted to do."

Jack and Barbara realized that the only way the girls would feel comfortable was if Jack more actively participated in the everyday custodial and play aspects of parenting. He began to play with them more, read to them, and put them to bed. Although the goodbyes didn't get easier right away, over time, the girls became more accustomed to the fact that their Mom sometimes went out at night, and Dad was there to take care of them and have fun with them. "My confidence in my husband's ability to take care of the kids increased and so did his, which made everything about my going out more pleasant," says Barbara.

WHEN NIGHTS OUT ARE DIFFICULT

Sometimes a combination of circumstances will conspire against your being able to have regular dates with your spouse. Rather than put your needs for time together on hold, you may be able to come up with a solution so that your relationship doesn't suffer.

Michael and Sarah Young (not their real names)

found it tough to go out when their children were 1½ and 3½. Both Betsy and Billy put up a big fuss when their parents left. Once his parents were gone, Billy would cry, then go to sleep until his parents returned, whether or not it was his nap- or bedtime. The psychologist they saw explained that Billy's hibernation was a coping response to separation, and that it was fine. It didn't seem to disrupt his sleeping patterns, so the Youngs didn't discourage the behavior.

"The psychologist encouraged us to go out on a date at least once every 2 weeks," says Sarah. "It helped me to hear her say that I had to teach them that I would leave and come back, and that each time we left, it would get easier. We decided the way we'd feel most comfortable doing that was to hire two sitters so that each child had someone available for cuddling and comfort. That enabled me to go out and have a good time." Once the children were another year older, having one sitter seemed to work fine. "I've come to realize that having difficulty saying goodbye is partly a function of a child's personality and partly part of growing up," says Sarah.

WHEN KIDS ARE STRESSED OUT

Like adults, children experience stress. And for children, several small things can contribute to a feeling of being overwhelmed. It may be that the usual routine at your house has recently been altered by a vacation, a business trip, extra-long work hours for you, or the arrival or departure of a house guest. Or it may be a bigger change, such as a marital separation, the death of a grandparent, or the arrival of a new sibling. When that's the case, your heading off for a date may precipitate a major goodbye protest or bad behavior while you're gone.

After the birth of their third daughter, Barbara Watson had an unnerving experience when she left all three girls (the older ones were 5 and 3) with a new sitter. Lana, the oldest, mooned the grandmotherly sitter and tried to push her down the steps. She also announced to the shaken sitter: "If my mom can't be here, I'll take care of my sisters myself."

Barbara was upset when she found out what had happened. "I had to reassure the sitter, who was in tears, and I had to lay down the law to my daughters. I told them I needed a few hours a week to myself and made it clear that no matter how awful they were, I was going to go," she says. It worked.

Finally, keep in mind that even when you've established a dating pattern, a relationship with a good sitter, or a smooth-sailing goodbye routine, your child may make a fuss about your leaving for no apparent reason.

Brette Tell never had problems with her mom or dad leaving her in the care of someone else until she was a few months past her fourth birthday. "When my husband and I were leaving the house one night to have dinner with a friend who came in from out of town, Brette went bananas," explains Phyllis Ruja Tell, her mother. "She started with delay tactics, like 'I want Mommy to make my bath. I want Mommy to take off my clothes.' I did it to placate her, but afterward she cried and hung on my leg as I tried to go out the door.

I cannot handle letting her cry; it reminds me of how upset I used to get when I was her age and my parents went out," explains Phyllis.

Phyllis and her husband, Frank, saw a family therapist who urged them to be reassuring but firm when they left and not to be taken in by Brette's last-minute requests to delay their departure. "It's still hard for me when Brette cries, but I know that she's going through a stage that will probably pass," says Phyllis. "She's in good hands, and she is able to have a good time with her sitter."

There's nothing wrong with calling home within a half-hour to make sure that your child has settled down. If the sitter reports that problems are continuing, offer some suggestions on what she might do to stop the crying or distract your child. And check in again. Chances are good that within the hour, all will be well, unless something more serious is going on. If the sitter has had experience caring for your child before, the problem may be that your child is coming down with a cold or just having a bad night for reasons that may never become apparent. (It will have to be your call whether to interrupt or shorten your evening out. You run the risk, however, of setting a dangerous precedent if you return home earlier than planned and your child is old enough to grasp the fact that he can get you to do it again by employing the same behavior tactics.)

If, however, the sitter has been with you only a few times, and each time you leave, tears or other inappropriate behavior continue, you may want to consider not using that sitter again. She may not be experienced enough to handle a child your child's age. Although it's an outside possibility, there's always the chance that she may be neglecting or not attending to your child's needs. If your child is not yet verbal and cannot answer simple questions such as, "What did you and Natasha play last night while Mommy and I were out?" you're probably better off finding a sitter who is more attentive to or skilled at handling your child. If your child ever volunteers information or answers your questions in a way that makes you suspicious or uncomfortable, talk to your sitter and get her version of events. (While there is likely to be some truth in what your child has said, he may have omitted important facts or put a spin on an event that gave you cause for concern than is unwarranted.) When in doubt, find another sitter.

Even if you conquer your fears about leaving your baby in someone else's care, convince yourself you deserve an outing, and hire the president of the local babysitter's club to sit for you on a regular basis, you may have one last hurdle to overcome: discovering that you simply hate to be away from your child.

Be firm with yourself—you, your partner, and your child will all benefit if you give yourself a break from time to time. Most parents still don't leave for a few hours without a few backward glances. Just remember that this reluctance to leave your children is perfectly natural—it's nature's way of making sure parents take care of their kids. Wanting to go out without them once in a while, however, is just as natural. So leave them in good hands, kiss them goodbye, and go!

✿ FOUR

When School
Bells Ring

Whether you decide to send your 2½-year-old to preschool several days a week or keep her at home until kindergarten, starting school is a big step. It may be your child's first real independent foray into the social world beyond your home and family, out of your sight and beyond your control. How easy or difficult the transition from home to school is for your child depends on a number of things, including:

- Age, both chronological and developmental
- Temperament
- Whether older siblings are already at school
- Whether your child will already know one or more classmates
- Your comfort or uneasiness about sending your child (if your own early experiences were unpleasant, you may inadvertently communicate your anxiety to your child)

- Whether there are any unusual stresses or changes at home (a move, a divorce, the impending arrival of another child)

Although it may seem at times like an overwhelming step to turn your child over to total strangers and separate from him several times a week or perhaps every day, going to preschool is in most children's best interest. It provides opportunities to learn the basics of following directions, playing cooperatively, and getting involved in activities that may not be available in the home (a gym, messy crafts), among other things.

Just as important is the lesson school teaches your child about goodbyes: Mommy or Daddy (or a trusted caregiver) can leave me in a different setting with other adults and kids and will come back to pick me up again. "Separating is a part of life, and it's just as important for children to learn how to be away from their parents as it is for them to learn their ABC's," says Dr. Stana Paulauskas.

READY OR NOT?

AGE FLAG: 2 TO 5 YEARS

Readiness is a word that gets used to describe a child's skills and developmental level, but it also involves whether a child is prepared to handle routine separations from family. In this section, you will find out more about what that means, and how you can help your child to feel comfortable making this important transition.

Preschools accept children at different ages, depending on the type of program they offer. Some offer parent and toddler programs for toddlers as young as 18 months, provided the parent or caregiver stays with the child. Others allow children to start at 2 or 2½, but may require that they be out of diapers. Still others focus on kindergarten preparation and accept children in the 1 or 2 years prior to their first year of kindergarten. Many of these include pre-K programs for children who are old enough for kindergarten but would benefit from another year of growth and socialization.

If you're a first-time parent, you will also probably have difficulty judging whether your child is ready to be away from home several hours a day without you or a trusted caregiver close at hand. "Even though children may be of a similar chronological age, they may be at very different developmental levels," explains Dr. Barbara Talent.

For example, one 3-year-old may be completely toilet-trained, able to express herself well verbally, and be able to confidently leave her mother's side to join a group of children playing in a sandbox in the neighborhood park. Another child the same age may still wear training pants, communicate her needs through pointing and pulling her mother by the sleeve to show her what she wants, and stay in her mother's lap when other children are playing close by. Despite the differences in their development, both children are normal—but the first is a more likely candidate to thrive in a preschool program than is the second.

Preschooler Readiness Checklist

Each preschool has its own requirements, but the following checklist of desirable preschool behaviors can help you decide if your child will be able to function well in a nursery school. The child:

* Can feed herself efficiently
* Is toilet-trained (some schools may not require this)
* Can express feelings—especially negative feelings—*appropriately*
* Understands that most things have their proper places
* Can control his impulses—he does not usually break away from you and dash into the street, grab things off the shelves of the grocery store, or hit or bite when angry
* Understands basic rules at home: do not run in the house, do not throw things, do not mistreat pets or other children
* Has interest in (and preferably some experience) playing with other children the same age
* Feels secure in her relationship with at least one adult (mother, father, or both) and has some other special adults—friends or relatives—who care for her and whom she loves

Are You Ready to Let Go?

Some parents decide to enroll their child in preschool because all the parents they know are signing up their kids (and who will their child play with if he does not also go?) Others simply want to do the right thing for their child, and preschool seems to be the accepted precursor to school. A few are fearful that unless they get their child in early, they won't be able to get into a highly competitive school at a later point.

In their hearts, however, some of these parents are deeply divided about whether they want their child to go because they remember how difficult early school experiences were for them.

"As a first-grader, I put my mother through the grinder because I did not want to go to first grade," says Louise Rogers, whose daughter Emma is now 6. "I remember refusing to get out of the car and generally being a pill about going. That's why I could relate so easily to Emma's belligerence about not going to preschool when she was almost 4."

It wasn't that Emma didn't have experience in preschool; she'd successfully completed a 3-day-a-week program the previous year. But out of the blue, she refused to go. After a week of "Mommy, I won't go," Louise enlisted the help of a teacher's aide who Emma loved. When it was time to say goodbye, the aide would hold the sobbing but compliant Emma on her lap. "The teachers told me she would cry for a while after I left, but they were patient with her, and the crying stopped after about a month," says Louise. "Even though I knew she would be fine, these few weeks were heartbreakers for me because the memories of my own reluctance about going to school were reignited," adds Louise.

"If you had problems with separation when you were little, watching your child go through something similar can awaken the emotions that you felt as a child," says Dr. Leslie Rescorla. "What's important is that you try not to be overprotective and make an effort to avoid communicating reluctance at letting your child go," she adds.

If you discover that goodbyes are hard for you and your child, console yourself with the thought that you can benefit from learning how to separate from your child. The year or more that your child spends in preschool is practice for that day when you have to pack your little one off to school. If both of you have successfully been able to navigate the ups and downs of preschool separations, then you will have developed a strong sense of trust in one another: your child knows that you will be there when he needs you, and you will come to realize that your child is secure enough in his attachment to you to enjoy what life has to offer him.

The amount of practice your child has had in separating from you is not always a determinant in how easy the adjustment to school will be, but it can be a factor. "We've found that 4-year-olds who have never before had someone other than Mom or a close relative caring for them have the most difficult time starting preschool," says Patricia Schindler, director of Newcomb Child Care Center of Tulane University in New Orleans. "They have built up an expectation about who will take care of them and they aren't used to being with strange adults," she says.

If you decide to keep your child at home because you cannot find a program you like or feel that your child is not ready, don't worry that your child will be at a disadvantage in kindergarten. "If you make the effort to ensure that your child has opportunities to separate from you and has opportunities to play with other children her age, she'll probably do fine," says

William Pfohl, Psy.D., professor of psychology at Western Kentucky University in Bowling Green.

If Your Child Doesn't Attend Preschool . . .

If you choose not to have your child attend preschool, consider doing one or more of the following on a regular basis so that your child gets practice being apart from you for short periods:

* Participating in a "Mother's day out" program (moms alternate caregiving to relieve each other)
* Putting your child in the nursery at your church or synagogue
* Hiring a sitter while you go out alone, with friends, or with your spouse
* Taking your child to playdates at friends' houses
* Joining a mother-and-child play group; even if you are present, your child will begin to practice separation as she gravitates toward play with the other children

EVALUATE A SCHOOL AND ITS GOODBYE POLICY

AGE FLAG: 2 THROUGH 5 YEARS

When you are looking for a school for your child, be sure to ask about how they handle goodbyes. What you learn is a good barometer of how child-oriented the school is and how the administration and staff view their relationship with you. A school's separation philosophy may be stated as formal policy on paper or may be more informal or even up to individual teachers (in which case it's smart to do some observing during a drop-off time).

Some schools do not want parents in the classroom (or simply do not have the space to accommodate them). If you suspect that goodbyes may be a problem for your child, this situation may prove unacceptable. Schools that are sensitive to children's needs are likely to take a number of steps to make sure children are ready to participate in class activities; they are often the same schools that encourage parents to stand by (if not in the classroom or hallway, then in a designated parent room) until their child adjusts to the routine of saying goodbye and going to school.

Schools whose teachers send notes to each incoming child or make a home visit before school bells ring are clearly tuned in to separation issues. So are those who invite the input of parents by asking them to describe what their child is like (personality traits, special skills and interests, potential behavior trouble spots, and changes at home that may have an impact on the transition to school).

✳

Find Out About a School's Goodbye Policy

While the way a school's goodbye policy isn't the only basis on which to select a school, it can be very important if daily contact with your child's teachers is important to you and you want to be sure your child isn't having adjustment problems. If possible, ask if you can visit at the beginning of the school day when parents are dropping off their children—it's the best way to see for yourself how teachers handle goodbye problems. Beyond that, find out:

* What is the policy of the school regarding separation at the beginning of the school year?
* Is there a "parents' room" where you or your child's caregiver is expected to stay "on call" during the first 1 or 2 weeks of school?
* Do parents escort their children to the preschool building, or are they allowed into the classroom?
* Are parents asked to leave by a particular time?
* Can you observe your child after you have bid him goodbye? (Some university preschools offer two-way observation rooms that parents are welcome to use.)
* Does the school encourage (or insist) on your staying with your child if he is having problems with your leaving? (And how do you feel about this?)
* How do teachers and staff handle children who are having problems with goodbyes?
* What does the teacher/school do if a child is having persistent and disruptive goodbye outbursts?
* Has the school ever had to ask a parent to withdraw a child due to separation difficulties?

Understanding the temperament of your child can help you make the important decision of whether a school's separation policy is likely to present a major problem or be a big help with goodbyes.

"My daughter Elise was the quintessential 'difficult child' who disliked change and a high level of stimulation," says Jeannette Beeger. "I also learned from organizing a play group that when I was one of the moms on duty, Elise clung to me. That made me realize that a preschool where there was no parent involvement would be best for her because she wouldn't be confused by both the stimulus of a new situation and not knowing when I'd leave," says Jeannette. She later chose a primary school whose policy it was to have parents drive up and drop off their child without setting foot on the school grounds. "For Elise, the more prolonged the goodbye, the longer her recovery, so the quick separation worked best for her," says Jeannette.

Knowing your child and being a good judge of whether the school is a good fit is critical. "If your child does not move into new situations or approach new children with ease, you want to make sure that the teachers have the capacity to recognize your child's need to approach things slowly and not be an overly controlling type who forces a child into play or conversation he's not ready for, however cheerfully it's done," says Dr. Talent.

Choosing a school that's the right match, in terms of both its goodbye policy and the program itself, isn't easy. And what works for the parents of one child with a sensitive temperament may not work for another. Cathie and Bob Schmidt decided to put their son, Andy, in nursery school 2 afternoons a week when he was 3. The school required parents to drop their child off (a teacher would take the child from the car in the morning and escort him back to his waiting parent when school was over). "Some days Andy pouted as he was taken; other days he'd kick, scream, and cry," remembers Cathie. "It really upset me, but I kept him in the whole year because the teachers told me that if I gave in and didn't make him come, he would think I wasn't in control. They had master's degrees in child development; I had a business degree, and Andy was my first child, so I believed them. Now, three kids later, I've learned that no one has dibs on what's right," says Cathie.

"Chances are good that this particular preschool was not a comfortable place for Andy," says Dr. Kathy Nathan. "Even children who have difficulty with transitions, however, can be otherwise 'ready' for school. Good programs and skilled teachers can figure out the comfortable way for temperamentally sensitive children to separate," she says.

Based on Andy's first and subsequent preschool experiences, Cathie and Bob decided to have Andy (who has a summer birthday) start kindergarten at age 6. They have not regretted their decision. "Andy is doing well in school, but he's still a very emotionally sensitive kid; even now, at 9, he looks over his shoulder and keeps me in view as long as he can as he walks to the school bus," says Cathie.

Visit and Evaluate Prospective Schools

Visiting a prospective school when the children and teachers are interacting is the best way to make an informed decision. You'll get a gut sense of whether it's the right environment for your child if you make the following observations and ask these questions:

- How do the teachers interact with the children? Do they get down on the children's level and make eye contact?
- Do the teachers and aides spend more time talking with the children than with each other?

- Do teachers adjust their interactions depending on the child? For example, does the teacher speak calmly and forcefully to children whose behavior is out of line? Does she make it a point to involve a child who does not seem to know what to do next in an activity or play group?
- Do teachers seem to be enjoying their work?
- Do you find the personalities and classroom style of the teachers appealing?
- How is discipline handled?
- Ask, "Do you use the same curriculum for all of the children?" The answer should reflect the fact that at least some of the lessons are tailored to the level and style of individual children.
- Ask, "What is a typical day like here?" This will give you some sense of the routine at transition times (dropping off and picking up) and clue you in about whether the amount of independence assumed for the children is right for your child ("Then each child goes to the bathroom as he finishes his art project before lunch" versus "Then we take the children to the bathroom and have them wash their hands for lunch.")
- Do you feel that your child would comfortably fit into the class and the school?

✳

PREPARE YOUR CHILD FOR SCHOOL

Probably the single best thing you can do is to attend an open house that's designed for parents and kids. Your child will get the chance to meet his teachers and see what his classroom and school building look like. Young children who lack sophisticated verbal skills can especially benefit from this in-person introduction to nursery school.

If you cannot attend with your child, find out if you can visit at another time. When my 3-year-old son Wil broke out with chicken pox 4 days before his preschool orientation, he was panic-stricken. His teachers invited us to visit the school after the other children had left, so he got a private guided tour (no one else got chicken pox!) When the blisters subsided and Wil was able to start school a week later, he was pleased to find himself something of a minor celebrity whom all the children were looking forward to meeting. So in spite of his recent illness, he had little trouble separating from us on his first day, in part because he didn't feel like he was going to an unfamiliar place.

AGE FLAG: 2 AND 3 YEARS

If your child is starting preschool at age 2 or 3, your first mention of the start of school need come no earlier than 1 or 2 weeks before the first day. Explain what's going to happen by saying, "Pretty soon you get to play at preschool. I'll go with you and we'll meet the teacher and other kids together."

AGE FLAG: 4 AND 5 YEARS

For a child of 4 or 5, you can and should begin talking about what your chid can expect at least a month beforehand. You might even want to do a calendar countdown if you sense your child is eagerly anticipating it.

If, on the other hand, you have the kind of child who gets anxious when he knows change is imminent, tread carefully. Four-year-old Sam Wolf grew more anxious with each discussion of the beginning of preschool, and frequently burst into tears. "I'm just not sure this preschool thing is a good idea," he told everyone who would listen. On his first day, he very reluctantly said goodbye to his parents, Tom and Janet. When Janet picked him up at the end of the day, however, he told his astonished and relieved mother, "Wow! Today was the greatest day of my life!"

What You Can Do Before School Starts

There are a number of other things you can do to help your child prepare for and be excited about starting nursery school. For a child between 2½ and 3 years old, it's best to do the following a week in advance. With older 3's and young 4's who are more skilled socially and have a better sense of time, you may want to start these activities 2 or 3 weeks in advance of the start of school.

* Find out if a class list with names and phone numbers is available 1 or 2 weeks prior to the start of school. Go over the names of the children with your child, and consider inviting over one or more children before school begins so your child will recognize a familiar face or two.
* Ask your librarian to recommend books or videos about starting school and read or view them with your child.
* Pick out some new clothes and select a special outfit for the first day (make sure that it's washable and your child knows it's okay to get paint or juice on it).
* If your child will take lunch or a snack to school, let

her help you choose a lunch box and plan a menu of lunches or snacks.

- Give your child something special to take with her to school. Many preschools discourage children from bringing toys. If you're not sure whether a stuffed animal will be frowned upon, give your child a photo of the two (or three of you) to keep in her lunch box or cubby.

THE FIRST WEEK OF SCHOOL

If school policy allows or encourages you to stay in the classroom or close by, find out what the teacher's expectations are about your role ahead of time. Ask where you should stand or sit, what you should or shouldn't do while you're there (escort your child to the bathroom, get her a class of water, assist her in getting out or putting away materials). The teacher may want you to be there but to keep your distance so your child learns he has to address the teacher and not you if he wants or needs something.

Even if the teacher seems open to your interacting with your child, keep in mind that you should not hover or do too much for your child. If your child says, "Mommy, I'm thirsty," you might reply, "I think there's a water fountain nearby. Why don't you ask Ms. Cohen if you can get a drink? She'll tell you where it is, and I'll be right here when you get back."

Make sure your child knows what to expect from you when you are in the classroom and when you leave. If you are staying, say so and tell him what you

are going to do. If you are getting ready to leave, let
him know that, too. Even if it looks as though your
child has gotten happily involved in a game with two
other children, and you hesitate to rock the boat, stopping by where he is playing for a kiss and a brief goodbye hug is a good idea. If you slip off while he is busy
with something else, he will have a hard time focusing
on an activity at drop-off time in the future for fear
that you will disappear when he isn't looking.

"A good teacher will help the child begin to structure her time on arrival," says Dr. Talent. And if you
clue her in that your child may be especially in need
of help in getting involved, she'll know to say: "Hi,
Paul! You're just the boy I need to pile up these blocks
for me—can you do that?" If, however, things are especially hectic or the teacher is busy with another
child, don't hesitate to help your child get involved
with either other children or an activity.

If your child is still crying a little when you leave,
don't be too concerned. "Usually children who act upset when their parents leave get over it quickly. If,
however, they see their parents look in through a classroom door or window, or even when they come to pick
them up after school, the crying may begin again,"
says Merle Marsh, head of the Lower and Middle
Schools at Worcester Country School in Maryland.
Linger around the corner within earshot or have another parent check out the classroom scene if you need
to be convinced your child is fine.

Most children settle into a happy enough routine of
such separations after just a few days, especially if the
teachers are warm and engaging and the activities are

varied and fun. There are always a few children, though, who continue to be reluctant to separate, even after several days of easing into the preschool routine.

Billy Young was one of them. As a 2-year-old, he did not have big troubles with goodbyes because he was in the same multi-age group preschool classroom as his sister, who is 17 months older. But when he returned to the same preschool a year later and Betsy went off to kindergarten, he would not leave his mother's side. "I felt as if I did preschool all over again," says Sarah. "I stayed with him from September until the Christmas holidays. Of course, when I was there, he would stay by my side." Although the teachers encouraged Sarah to continue to stay (it was their philosophy that a parent should stay as long as the child "needed" them), she finally couldn't take it anymore. "I told them I'd wait in the screening room (where there's a one-way mirror that allows parents to watch what's going on without the children seeing them) until he settled down." The head teacher carried him around while he cried for 20 minutes the first day, and less and less on subsequent days. Within a week's time, Sarah could leave so long as Billy was comfortably situated close to his favorite teacher.

If you know from past experiences with your child (being unable to leave a children's birthday party because he demands your presence) that goodbyes are likely to be an issue, you may want to make a school's goodbye policy a bigger factor in your decision about where to send your child than most parents do. Or if you know that a school or teacher is going to encourage you to stay, talk with the teacher or director about developing a strategy that will work not only for your child but for you, too.

Disengagement Strategies

If your child continues to act out when you say goodbye after you've had 1 or 2 weeks to practice perfecting your routine, try these disengagement strategies:

- Get advice from the teacher, who has no doubt had experience dealing with clinging vines, criers and screamers. You won't feel as conflicted when you leave after following what the two of you have agreed is a smart script. Most teachers are amenable to getting a check-in phone call once you arrive back home or at your office.
- If your child refuses to get out of the car or come into the building, talk to the teacher. He may be willing to cajole, reason with, or pick up and carry your child. If he cannot leave the classroom (or it's not safe to leave your child alone), just stand or sit for a few minutes (to refresh your frazzled nerves). Your child may change his mind.

    If that does not produce the desired result, be matter of fact about what you expect your child to do. Do not indulge your child's pleas to skip school, or you will end up reinforcing his behavior. Instead, stress how competent he is at getting dressed, playing on the computer, or riding his bike, and tell him that you're confident that he's big enough and brave enough to go to school.

If he's still unwilling to go, pick him up and carry him in. Again, stay as calm as you can even if he kicks or hits. Go through your goodbye routine as best you can. Then leave. It's unlikely his behavior will continue for long, since the audience he was acting out for (you) is gone. Again, if it will make you feel better, call the school and ask for a progress report when you get home or to the office.

Lorraine Bakke, a veteran kindergarten teacher, suggests that parents of children of kindergarten age or older who protest staying in school consider a "go home, no fun" strategy. Allow your child to return home (if that's an option for you) with the proviso that he not be allowed to play with his toys, watch TV, or play outside—in essence, he will have "nothing to do" for whatever period of time you can handle (since you must enforce the no-fun rule). This can be persuasive in his asking to return to school within an hour or two or in not pulling his usual "I won't go" routine in the future.

- Make sure your child knows that bad behavior will not get her what she wants. "Don't be afraid to tell your child that she must stop," advises Dr. Carol Seefeldt. "Her acting out may be her way of asking you to set limits. If you don't set them or you act like a child yourself by getting angry or making threats, your child will not learn to trust herself or become independent," she says.
- If your child tries to keep you at school by making a constant string of requests ("Come in the classroom and see the new fish, Mama. Now come and help me get my sitting mat out. Will you read this

story book to me?"), be firm and stick to your routine. If that is to allow your child to show you one
thing, stand your ground and conclude your goodbye
routine when your child makes his "stay here" pitch.

- If your child clings to you and has to be pulled off
  by a teacher, try this strategy: spend play time with
  your child when the two of you are physically close
  but not touching. "It's a way of modeling closeness
  that's not clinging, and it will be easier for you to
  set limits and enforce them when it comes time for
  goodbyes," says Dr. Julia Robertson. Also, know
  that it's okay for a teacher to peel your clinging vine
  from you, even if he screams and flails. Tell him you
  love him, that you'll see him after lunch, and go. "If
  you don't try to stop the clinging behavior, you are
  sending the message to your child that she can manipulate you with her behavior," says Dr. Robertson.
  "And the appropriate message to send is, 'You can't
  always get what you want.'"

- If you and your child have entered an escalating
  cycle of anger, tears, and frustration over goodbyes
  at school, try having someone else drop your child
  off. A spouse is a natural first candidate, if his or her
  schedule permits. A grandparent, familiar caregiver,
  or any other adult the child knows well and feels
  comfortable with are all possibilities—but realize
  that you will still have to re-establish a workable
  goodbye routine if you are going to resume taking
  your child to school.

- Resist your urge to overprotect your child by giving
  in on a goodbye issue. "Children have to learn to
  deal with the darts and arrows of life," says Dr.

Seefeldt, "and in helping your child to get through a difficult goodbye, you are helping him develop competence."

Keep in mind that most bad goodbye behavior ends shortly after you and your child separate. But do talk to your teacher to confirm whether your child continues to cry or misbehave once you've gone. If she quiets down quickly and engages in the activities of the day, you should be able to change the departure behavior if you stick to your goodbye ritual and hang tough on not tolerating inappropriate behavior. If, however, the teachers reports that your child continues to show her distress in ways that are disruptive to others or to her participation and enjoyment of the school day, ask for their advice in what you as a team should do. And be open to the idea of getting professional help (the particulars are described in Chapter Two on page 59).

When There's Backsliding

Children who have taken longer than their classmates to make the transition to school are susceptible to returning to bad goodbye behavior. The reasons may be events in your child's life that, while they may not seem like a big deal for you, are just enough to throw her. Returning to school after having been on vacation, suffering from an illness (however minor), or having grandparents or other relatives stay with your family can precipitate a goodbye crisis.

Backsliding can also occur if your child is developing a new skill. "Periods of regression are the norm for young children," says Dr. Robertson. "When they're focusing their efforts on a new cognitive or motor area, they feel challenged and taxed, which often means they'll regress emotionally," she says. The catalyst for backsliding with goodbyes can also be something that's happened at school—for example, having a favorite teacher or classmate leave.

A change in the daily routine at school caused 3½-year-old Amy Shevchik to insist that her mother, Leigh Ann, carry her into the school, which represented a return to earlier separation difficulties. "When she started going to her new school, I carried her into the classroom, a practice I soon discovered made good-byes much worse because she clung to me," explains Leigh Ann. "Once I recognized that, I stopped doing it and made our goodbyes very orderly, which she responded to well. But when spring came and we arrived to find her classmates outside at play instead of inside the classroom, it threw her off."

Leigh Ann solved the backsliding problem by agreeing to carry Amy to the classroom, where they deposited her lunch in her cubby and her feet on the floor. The first week, Amy grabbed hold of her mother's legs and walked behind her to the play area. But during the next 2 weeks, Amy agreed to hold her mother's hand and walk beside her. Once a teacher or one of Amy's classmates came over to her, she had no problem saying goodbye to her mother. "I knew I couldn't give in and carry her to the playground because she's more dependent on me if I'm holding her," says Leigh Ann. "And with some encouragement, she did respond to my telling her that she was a big girl and capable of walking to the playground by herself."

Because other parents witnessed the difficulties Amy had with goodbyes both at the beginning of school and 6 months later, they offered Leigh Ann lots of advice on how to handle it. So did her pediatrician and her therapist. "In the end, I discovered that what was most important was to tune in to my child's personality and what felt comfortable to me. Giving her some choices about things, all of which were acceptable to me, helped the two of us establish a routine that worked for us," she says.

STRESS CAN PRECIPITATE A GOODBYE CRISIS

Even children who had no goodbye problems when they started preschool are not immune to experiencing some farther down the road. Three-year-old Laura Watson parted easily from her mother Barbara during her first 2 weeks at preschool. But the goodbye protests began during week 3, just before Barbara gave birth to her third child. "Her teacher would have to restrain her so that I could leave the classroom," says Barbara. After the birth of her sister, Laura continued to beg her father, who took over the job of dropping her off, not to leave her. "Laura didn't want to even go to school because she said she didn't want to be away from the baby, but I know that it was because she wanted to be with me," says her mother. Barbara worked out a plan with Laura's teacher; they decided that Barbara would stay for 15 minutes, then leave, no matter how much Laura protested. "It took a week to make her realize that I was going to go, no matter what she did," says Barbara. "And after that, she was fine."

While the birth of a new sibling often precipitates a

goodbye crisis (or some other behavioral reaction), other events can have the same effect on goodbyes, including an impending business trip that you or your spouse must take, a favorite sitter leaving, or marital difficulties, particularly separation or divorce. These and other events can result in your child feeling anxious about having you leave him, even if his adjustment to school has been smooth up until this point.

Four-year-old Eric Schmidt broke down in tears when his mother Sue dropped him off at preschool during a short period when she was undergoing medical testing. "I wasn't sure what was wrong with me, and although I didn't discuss it with Eric, he knew I wasn't feeling like my old self and must have picked up on the fact that I was worried," says Sue. So she and Eric's teacher went back to the goodbye ritual that had helped many of Eric's classmates part from their parents at the beginning of the school year: to wave goodbye to the parting parent through the "goodbye window" while being held or comforted by the teacher. "When I disappeared from view, Eric would recover, and once the tests showed that there was nothing seriously wrong with me (which made me feel less anxious), Eric went back to his usual 'See you, Mom' when I dropped him off," says Sue.

When you talk to your child's teacher about things that are going on at home that may be affecting goodbyes, you need not reveal details about your personal life that you'd prefer to keep private, but share enough so that he will have an insight into what's behind the suddenly difficult goodbyes. Ask for his help in engaging your child so that you can leave without a scene.

When a separation or divorce is happening to a family, it's particularly important to work with your child's school (or daycare center) to minimize drop-off and pick-up problems. "It's important for both parents to carefully work out the arrangements so that there's no mix-up about who is picking up the child," says Patricia Schindler. "The more consistent you can be about the days or times when either parent is picking up the child, the better. It's one less confusion for the child during a time of family turmoil," she says.

No matter what the stress, you might want to give some thought to whether you can reduce your child's anxiety by being more available to your child when he's not in school, rescheduling a vacation or trip so that it comes at a less stressful time, or by acknowledging your child's feelings and reassuring her that you will always be there for her.

UNDERSTANDING OCCASIONAL SEPARATION BLUES

Once your child settles into the routine of preschool, separations will get easier, but that doesn't mean you should never expect a problem. It is perfectly normal for a child to go through periods during which she suddenly has trouble separating or is misbehaving in school for no apparent reason. Here are a number of common scenarios and how to handle them:

- *Morning foot-dragging.* As an adult, you've certainly had days when you would have preferred to sleep in, call in sick, or let your responsibilities slide. Children have days like this, too. Dr. Nathan urges parents to avoid power struggles with children on mornings like these. "Arguing and reasoning can be futile. Just say, 'All of us have bad days, and I'm sorry you feel that way this morning.'"

You can defuse a lot of morning battles, and sometimes even head them off before they begin, by letting your child make choices (all of which are acceptable to you) about what she wears, which stuffed animal she takes to school, what to have for breakfast, or which route to take to school. "The more choices you give children, the better," says Dr. Seefeldt. "It gives them a feeling of being in control, and helps them to develop competence," she adds.

- *"Why do I have to go to preschool?"* Resist the urge to justify your whole life style to your child. You don't need to get into long discussions of your personal or economic need for employment, or for some child-free time to pursue your own interests, or the benefits you hope she will get out of attending preschool. Just keep it simple and understandable. "Everyone has their job. My job is to work in an office (or to take care of the family and the house) and your job is to go to preschool" should suffice. Make sure your child knows that attending school is a given, that she has no choice in the matter, and you will avoid a lot of argument. If you get a lot of resistance about school attendance, concentrate on what is going to happen after school: "Oh, don't forget, today's the day we're going apple picking after school."

- *Misbehavior at school.* When a child is feeling insecure or anxious, acting out may be his way of expressing it. Talk to the teacher about how she is handling the situation at school and let your child know that you are aware of what he did. Acknowledge his feelings ("I know that it's hard for you to say goodbye to Mom in the morning"), but tell him what's not acceptable ("But you can't knock over the other children's buildings just because you're mad that I left"). When you hear from the teacher that your child has changed his bad behavior, tell him how pleased you are.

- *Late pickups.* Few school experiences are more frightening for a child than being the last one to be picked up. Keep in mind that even 5 minutes can seem like an eternity to a child. Try to come a moment or two early every day, so that you are already there the first time your child thinks to check the crowd of waiting parents for your face. The younger your child, the more important it is to be on time. If you must be late, let the school know or try to make arrangements for another person who your child knows to pick her up.

- *Musical chairs pickup.* If there is no predictable routine to who is picking up your child, he may become anxious about goodbyes and pickups. You can reduce it by reminding you child as you drop him off who to look for when school is over. If your child is sensitive to changes in routine, make sure that everyone who takes him to and from school follows the same drop-off ritual: taking the same route, going in the same door, hanging up knapsack and jacket, greeting the teacher, getting involved in an activity, and saying goodbye.

- *Loss of bladder control.* Occasional toileting accidents even in children who are well trained are very common among preschoolers, especially at the beginning of the year. While such episodes may contribute to your child's reluctance to have you leave, it doesn't mean that your child isn't ready for school. He may be having trouble isolating the bodily feelings that tell him he needs to go to the bathroom from the stimulation of a roomful of noisy children. In addition, he may be nervous about unfamiliar places like the school bathroom, which probably seems larger and louder and generally more intimidating than the one at home. Throw in his need to ask people who are still virtual strangers for help with intimate tasks like zipping up his fly, and you have a sure-fire recipe for occasional accidents.

A good preschool teacher will not make much of these lapses (or allow the other children to), but will matter-of-factly help children on with their spare clothes. You can help by being just as nonchalant about what happened, by dressing your child in clothing she can pull on and off by herself (elastic-waist jeans, for instance, are a better choice than overalls or pants with snaps and zippers), and praising her when she has gone a long time without having an accident.

WHAT'S BEHIND DIFFICULT GOODBYES

Your child's reluctance about going to school may not be a separation problem, but something that is happening at school. It's usually best to take a less-than-direct approach and ask your child what she likes and doesn't like at school. She may say that a particular child is making fun of her or excluding her from play. If that's the case, talk to the teacher and ask him to monitor the situation and intervene as needed.

Another possibility is that your child may be concerned about a task at school that he doesn't feel up to. Many boys lag behind girls in their fine-motor skill development and may find activities that involve using scissors or crayons so difficult or their skills so lacking that they want to avoid them altogether. Again, getting the teacher's input and help here is critical.

The problem may be the teacher herself. Your child and the teacher may simply not "click." Your child may pick up on the fact that the teacher doesn't like him or is "mean" to him. Or you may observe it yourself during pickup and drop-off times. At schools where there is more than one class of children of a particular age, you may be able to request a transfer. If your child is balking about going to school because of the teacher, and you have observed that their relationship is not what it should be, don't hesitate to request a different teacher out of fear of being branded an interfering parent. Follow your instincts and do what's best for your child. If transferring to another class is not a possibility, investigate other programs. If you find a setting and teacher you feel is more appropriate, and the situation at school has remained unchanged, seriously consider making the change.

Peggy Tabacco quickly zeroed in on the fact that her son Ted's preschool teacher was not the kind of warm, responsive teacher that she wanted for her 3-year-old. "I was appalled that she had a set of headphones on in the morning, as the children were coming into the classroom, and so were other parents," says Peggy. "But what really griped me was that she never smiled or laughed or seemed to enjoy her job."

At first, Peggy was reluctant to complain to the

school director about the teacher. But after a disagreement with the teacher over a particular goodbye one day (Ted was in tears and the teacher ordered Peggy to leave the classroom), she enlisted the support of other parents, who subsequently met with the school director and founders. "Shortly thereafter, we saw some changes in the teacher. The headphones came off, she smiled more often, and was more receptive to working with the parents on problems with their kids," says Peggy.

No matter how much effort you and your child's teacher may put into making goodbyes smooth and preschool fun, sometimes things just don't work out. Dr. Nathan describes the case of a 3-year-old child who cried not only when her mother left, but throughout the day. The child's mother had recently separated from her husband, moved back in with her parents, started school, and enrolled her child in nursery school, all within the space of a few months. The changes were more than the child could handle, so the mother wisely decided to take her daughter out of preschool and have her grandmother watch her while she attended classes.

Constant crying or other signs of stress that teachers point out should be taken seriously. Like this mother, you may need to search beyond goodbye tears to determine whether your child can comfortably handle being away from you and her home for hours or even a whole day. If there are no family problems that may be affecting your child's sense of security (as was true in the case described by Dr. Nathan), rethink whether preschool is the right place for your child right now. Be sure to talk to people who can help you to make an informed decision about whether to take your child out of school, or whether to consider another option like reducing the number of hours or days in the program, or whether another program might be more appropriate. Your child's teacher, the director of the preschool program, a child psychologist, and other parents can share their advice on this subject.

A year or more at school will leave most children feeling more at ease with predictable separations and more confident in their own budding social and cognitive skills. Though you may not believe it on the first tearful day of school, a week after summer vacation begins, you will probably hear your child say wistfully, "I sure do miss going to school!"

🎋 FIVE

Vacations and
Business Trips

Figuring out how to negotiate routine separations is challenging, particularly if your child has the kind of temperament that makes her sensitive to change. But finessing days, not hours, away from your child can be *very* difficult, particularly when you or your spouse has no choice in the matter because a trip is necessitated by work. Even when the separation is voluntary—a vacation with your spouse—your anticipation of romantic, uninterrupted meals, sleeping in or sleeping through the night, and hours of doing whatever you please is likely to be tempered by your concern for how well your child will cope in your absence. Because the demands of being a parent often steal energy and time from a couple's relationship, going on vacation is often the best way for a couple to recharge.

Still, many couples put it off because they worry about how their child will fare without them. What they don't realize, however, is that parents who don't allow themselves a break aren't doing their children any favors. "If you're under stress, putting off a vacation can be a mistake," says Dr. Barbara Talent. "Most harmful of all is the parent who is wound up in her own problems and isn't interacting enough with her child," she says.

Whether you feel you can handle being away from your child is an important consideration if the trip is optional rather than a necessity. While mothers are often thought to be more hesitant about leaving their child behind, fathers can be just as reluctant. When Marianne and Steve Johnston (not their real names) left their 15-month-old daughter Andrea for the first time, they decided to spend only 2 nights of a 3-day weekend away so they'd have 1 free day with her. "It was harder for Steve to leave her than it was me because he works long hours, and weekends are usually his only time to be with her," says Marianne, who is a full-time mother.

A full-time mother who is a veteran of holding down the fort during her husband's business trips, Joan Harlem decided that she needed a respite from constant caregiving, and arranged a 4-day trip with several friends from college. "When you are the parent who is at home a lot with your children while your spouse travels, you cannot afford to forget your own needs. I was feeling burned out, and this trip made me remember what it felt like to be independent again," says Joan. "It also made me feel very fortunate for what I have," she adds.

With the right preparation and support, your going away for several days can be a positive experience for your child. "Growing up means learning to deal with stress and change, and parents have to present appropriate opportunities for their child to learn to cope with both," says Dr. Talent.

AGE-BY-AGE REACTIONS

AGE FLAG: NEWBORN TO 6 MONTHS

Getting a handle on how your child will react to being apart from you for several days or even longer will depend once again on his developmental age. If your baby is 6 months old or younger, she is less likely to miss you than to notice that the person caring for her isn't as finely attuned to her needs as Mom and Dad are. Dr. Martha Farrell Erickson stresses that the during the first half of the first year, children should not be particularly disturbed by short separations from one parent or the other, as long as their caregiving situation remains fairly uniform.

AGE FLAG: 6 MONTHS TO 2 YEARS

After 6 months of age, babies begin developing the concept of object permanence—simply put, the ability to remember an object that the baby can no longer see, smell, taste, or hear. (Remember the ball-under-the-sofa example.) "We hypothesize that babies do the same with people, that when Mommy or Daddy says bye-bye, there is still a memory of the person," says Marilyn Montgomery, Ph.D., founder of the Wellspring Center for Family Development in Lubbock, Texas. The better able a child grasps the idea that when you go way, you'll come back, the easier it will be to cope with your being away for several days.

Although all young children feel the pain of separations keenly, long separations are probably the most difficult for children between about 8 months to 2 years of age. By this time, children have developed a marked fear of separation from their parents. To make matters worse, children of this age lack a good sense of time.

Making periodic short trips while your child is young is nonetheless a good idea. "Try to get away for at least a weekend by the time your child is 18 months old," recommends Dr. Janine Wenzel Reed. "If you postpone it until your child is older, it will probably be a bigger production for both of you than it need be," she adds. You can read more on how to make things easier for your child when you're away in the sections "Maintain the Routine" (page 134) and "While You're Gone" (page 135).

AGE FLAG: 2 TO 3 YEARS

Another characteristic of toddlers that affects their capacity to understand long separations is their inability to view things, whether events or actual physical objects, from another person's perspective. Psychologists call this egocentrism. A 3-year-old, for instance, may look at a page in his picture book and ask you, "What's this?"—unaware that you cannot see what he's looking at from across the room. Similarly, a 2-year-old may select a teddy bear for her father's birthday present because that is what she herself would like to receive.

When young children experience events that they cannot understand, egocentrism causes them to interpret things in terms of themselves. A 2½-year-old who is scolded for something in the morning and who falls down and cuts her knee in the afternoon may assume that she fell down because she had misbehaved in the morning. Similarly, if a parent is away for a long time, the child may blame herself for the parent's absence. She may tell herself, "Mommy's gone on a trip because I haven't been a good girl."

AGE FLAG: 4 TO 5 YEARS

Preschoolers are much better equipped to handle one or both of you being away for two reasons: they understand that you will come back if you leave, and they have presumably had positive experiences being cared for by other adults. Even children of this age, however, require reassurance and openings for them to express their sadness at the idea of your being gone. Five-year-old David Howell appeared content as he watched his mother pack for a 3-day business trip. When she started to pack the bag containing the knitting that she worked on while traveling, though, he suddenly snatched the tape measurer out of her bag. "You're taking this with you? I love this!" he cried, and burst into tears. David had no interest in his mother's tape measurer, but since he seemed to fix on it as a symbol of her departure, she decided it was more important to leave it with him than to take it with her. "Will you take good care of it for me?" his mother asked. David nodded and smiled, and ran to put the tape measurer on the table beside his bed.

Temperament Tales

Just as your child's temperament is a factor in routine separations, it will also influence how he reacts to lengthier separations. If you have the type of child who is sensitive to change, it's wise to assume that while you're gone, the less change in her routine, the better. She will also probably require more reassurance from you both before and after your trip.

"Alex is 6 now, but his pattern of getting upset when I have to go on a business trip has not changed since he was old enough to let me know how sad it made him feel when I left," says Tom Schmidt, a professor in the microecology department at Michigan State University. When Alex accompanied his mother and younger brother to the airport to see Tom off, his eyes teared up and he said, "Dad, when I grow up I'm going to be a scientist so I can go with you on your trip." Tom said, "I let him know that it's okay to feel sad, and tell him that I'm going to miss him, too. If it's early enough, I always call when I get there and tell them what the plane ride was like," says Tom.

As is the case with other goodbyes, the more ambivalent you are about leaving, the more likely it is that your child will pick up on your anxiety. So whether you're worried about the trip because you don't really enjoy visiting a new city on business, traveling by plane, or the prospect of leaving your child even though your spouse has been lobbying for the two of you to get away, try your best not to let it surface in your words, actions, or behavior.

Adjusting to Regular Trips

Another factor is how predictable and frequent your going away is. Tiffany Field, Ph.D., a professor in the

University of Miami Medical School's departments of pediatrics, psychology, and psychiatry, has studied the effects of mothers' business trips on their young children. She found that the first time or two that a child's mother was away, the child typically demonstrated her unhappiness through sleep disturbances (for instance, night waking in a child who had been sleeping through the night) and regression—that is, temporarily losing control of skills she had mastered (for example, potty training) or behaving as if she were younger (for example, using baby talk). When business trips occur regularly, however, children adjusted. "Kids become accustomed to them, and don't react as negatively over time," she explains.

Joan and Robert Harlem have gotten Robert's frequent, and sometimes lengthy, trips away down to a science. Robert is an attorney and must often conduct a trial in another city. "Robert is very aware that his being away has a major impact on Jonathan, who is 6, and Christopher, who is 4," says Joan, who is a full-time mom. "He's particularly sensitive to how they feel because his own father traveled extensively and didn't have much time to play with Robert."

Robert has a special ritual based on his special nicknames for his sons, "Jelly Bean" and Peanuts." When the boys wake up on mornings when Daddy's away, Jonathan finds a jelly bean under his pillow and Christopher finds a peanut. "We tell them it's Daddy's special fairy who delivered it because he was thinking of them. Jonathan is getting a little suspicious about who really puts it there, but both of them look forward to finding it, and it is a good reminder of Dad," says Joan.

WHEN TO BREAK THE NEWS . . . AND HOW

AGE FLAG: NEWBORN TO 2 YEARS

Getting your child used to the idea that you are going to be gone for a longer time than usual is critical to a successful transition. Explaining that you're going away to children under the age of 2 is difficult; still, child-development experts say that explaining what's going to happen in simple language in a reassuring tone goes a long way. Infants are acute perceivers of tension and anxiety, so try to be warm, relaxed, and confident when you talk to your baby about your departure. Babies as young as 11 months can understand simple sentences such as, "Mommy and Daddy are going bye-bye. Grandma will take care of you."

For toddlers, it's best to wait until the night before you leave to mention your plans. Don't go into a lot of detail or make a big deal out of it. But do try to link your departure to concrete events in the child's life that he will understand. "After breakfast tomorrow morning, Mom is going to be going away for a few days. Daddy will put you to bed for 2 nights, then Mom will be home again."

AGE FLAG: 3 TO 5 YEARS

It's better to alert your preschooler several days in advance of your leaving so that she has time to get used to the idea and ask questions about things that will affect her. A 4- or 5-year-old will be able to handle even more details. You might say, "I've got to go out of town to do some work next week, and I'll be gone for 3 days. Daddy will be here at night and in the mornings, and he will drop you off at daycare just like Mommy does with you every day. I'm going to Boston. It's the city we read about in *Make Way for Ducklings*. Come on, let's go see if we can find Boston on our map."

Again, relating things to your child's schedule will make it easier for her to understand. Providing a 3-year-old with a way to mark the passage of time while you're gone can be helpful. Give your child's caregiver candy to be given out after a particular meal on each day of your absence, and tell her "I will be home on the day you eat the last piece." Colored stones or marbles that can be moved from one basket to another can serve a similar function. A 4- or 5-year-old will probably find it comforting to know how to do a countdown so he can measure how soon you will be leaving, how long you will be gone, and when you'll be returning. You might buy special stickers for her to put on a calendar. If you're doing a countdown, however, make sure that business demands won't interfere with your intended date of return. Breaking a promise (even if it's beyond your control) is a sure-fire way to make your child distrustful of you.

It's wise to avoid discussing future plans within earshot of your child before you know they're going to happen and when. Children have good ears and powerful imaginations, and when they hear snippets of conversation with words like *travel, leaving,* and *when I'm gone,* in them, they fill in the missing details for themselves. The explanations he makes up may be far scarier than the reality. If your child tunes into the fact that you are leaving before you have made your formal announcement, be truthful. But you don't need to offer more information than she wants until closer to the time that you must leave.

When she hears your news, your child may react by explicitly telling you that she doesn't want you to go, or acting it out. When Dawn Basel (not her real name) told her 4-year-old daughter Lynn that she and Lynn's dad were going on vacation, Lynn replied: "I don't want you to go," and then asked if she could come along in her mother's suitcase. Lynn later fell asleep in her mother's suitcase as she was helping her pack. "It's normal for kids to get upset when parents are saying goodbye, but if I had a choice between a kid who screamed his lungs out and one who didn't react, I'd happily choose the screamer," says Dr. Byron Egeland.

Finally, don't make your trip sound like too much fun. Instead, focus on what your child will be doing while you are away.

Predeparture Behavior

It's not unusual for your child and you to experience some predeparture separation pangs. "When the parent is getting ready to leave, she often withdraws emotionally to protect herself from feeling guilty or sad, and her child can pick on that," says Dr. Montgomery. If your mind is on details related to the trip you're about to take, you can't be fully attentive to your child, either. When this happens, your child may feel that you have in some ways left him already, which may make him act out in some way—by doing irritating things to get your attention, pouting, or even unpacking your suitcase.

The day that Peggy Tabacco was leaving on a 5-day business trip, her 6-year-old son and 5-year-old daughter bickered with each other more than usual, and there seemed to be no end to their requests for her to play with them or help them with one thing or another. "I was sitting at my computer putting together a few last notes for a business meeting the next day when my daughter came in and threw herself on my desk. She was trying to get my attention, but she managed to smash my contact lenses that I'd put on my mouse pad because my eyes hurt," Peggy remembers. She didn't have an extra set, and getting another pair before she left wasn't possible. "I just lost it. I told my husband to watch the kids, then I went out into the backyard and had a good cry. I was upset about the lenses, of course, but I was also feeling on edge because I was about to leave my kids," says Peggy.

It's not unusual for parents to feel that way, according to Dr. Robertson, and edginess reflects a parent's guilt about having to leave. "It's critical to remind yourself that you cannot nurture your child unless you are taking care of your own needs, whether they're personal or professional," she says. "Once you make a decision to take a trip, let go of your angst so that you can use your emotional resources to help your child cope with your upcoming absence."

To the extent that it's possible, organize your work or your packing so that you can spend time with your child before you have to rush off. It's not unusual for children to act out before you leave; it's their way of expressing their unhappiness at your having to go. But if you can give them your attention and give them a few choices of things you can do together before you have to leave, you can help facilitate a smoother goodbye.

Maintain the Routine

Several factors affect how comfortable your child will feel about your not being with her. The most important is her familiarity with the person or people who are taking care of her. Grandparents and other relatives with whom your child has frequent contact are good bets; so are regular sitters. Ann Carson (not her real name) had her full-time sitter report to work at her parents' home when she and her husband went away because her 9-month-old was more used to her sitter's arms than she was her grandmother's. Using regular sitters to supplement your relatives' caregiving can also save wear and tear on everyone's patience, particularly if your child is at a demanding age or acts out while you're gone.

Having your sitter stay at your home is preferable to taking your child elsewhere, even if it's a grandparent's home, because it contributes to a sense of normalcy. If you have more than one child, it's much better to keep them together—having each other's company can be very reassuring—than to ship them off to different relatives. If you travel often, try to make the same caregiving arrangements for your child each time you are away; that in itself will make your leaving less traumatic.

If your child is attending school or participating in a play group, it's smart to continue that routine as well. "We found that kids whose parents were away did better if they stayed in nursery school, instead of having the mother arrange for someone like their grandmother or a substitute caregiver to take care of the child at home. The more closely you maintain your child's daily routine, the more predictability and stability she will experience, which should help her cope until you return," says Dr. Field. If it is at all possible, arrange for your child to be taken care of in your home—having friends or relatives care for her in their home may be more convenient for them, but it will be one more change for your child to cope with.

Regardless of who takes care of your child, it is a good idea to familiarize him or her with your child's schedule and preferences; even if your spouse is putting in more time on duty, share details he may not be aware of if he usually has a more limited caregiving role. It's best to write everything down: times when she is due to arrive at preschool, a prearranged playdate, or ballet class and directions on how to get there; times when she should be fed or given a bottle, put down for a nap, and bedded down for the night; the kinds of food she prefers and what you will and won't allow at various mealtimes and for snacks; and rules and routine's she's expected to follow (nightly baths morning and evening teeth brushing, picking up her toys in the morning before she goes to daycare). Whoever is taking care of your child can still expect to hear plenty of "That's not the way Mom (or Daddy) does it," but the more the "substitute you" follows your instructions, the less protest is likely.

While You're Gone

Even the best-behaved child may not act like herself when you're gone. The stress of Mommy or Daddy or both being away may be simply more than your child can handle, no matter what lengths you go to minimize the impact on her life.

Be sure to talk to your teacher and the person who will be caring for her about the possibilities. Sleep problems are common. Your child may be unable to fall sleep or stay asleep without someone staying with her, wake up in the middle of the night and call out, or experience bad dreams. One of the most gut-wrenching things for Lisa Forchay was that her 21-month-old daughter Whitney had nightmares about being attacked again by a dog (whose bites in real life had resulted in 30 stitches and plastic surgery on her face and ear) *only* when Lisa was away on business trips. "My husband would tell me that she'd scream out 'Bad doggy, bad doggy,' in her sleep," says Lisa. "It made me feel guilty and helpless, but once my husband was aware that it could happen, he at least felt prepared."

Regressive behaviors are another common reaction. If your child begins sucking his thumb again, has toileting accidents, or reverts to crawling once she's learned to walk, be sure to tell the caregiver not to tease, punish, or reprimand the child. What these behaviors signal is that your child is having a hard time coping with Mom or Dad or both being gone. If the skill is newly acquired, a regression isn't so serious. "It takes a lot of energy to keep a new skill going, energy that's often diverted to handling the stress of a parent not being around," says Dr. Talent. A cuddle and soothing comments about when Mom and Dad are coming back will probably provide the comfort that's needed. If a well-established skill doesn't come back within days of your return, however, you may want to consult your pediatrician or a child psychologist for ideas on how to handle the situation.

Children do not always show sadness as clearly as adults do. Irritability, an inability to get involved in play, and even being quieter than usual are all ways in which young children express sadness. An infant may sleep more than usual, or babble less. A 3-year-old may be listless or restless, and a 5-year-old may declare that he is bored and has no appetite.

What can be more problematic is a child who vents his anger at one or both parents' leaving by misbehaving at home or at school. When Bob Schmidt went on a business trip, 5-year-old Andy acted out. "He wouldn't get dressed for school, sit down for meals, or go along in any way with our routine," remembers Cathie. "He was my first child, and my response was to spank him or give him a time-out, which would escalate into a horrible scene because he refused to take the time-out. Now I realize that his acting out was his way of showing how emotionally out of sorts he felt when his dad left, so now I try to acknowledge his feelings. I give him art materials so he can express it that way or make something to give to his dad when he returns," says Cathie.

When Frank Tell and Phyllis Ruja Tell were on their first extended vacation, an 11-day trip to Europe, their 7-year-old son became aggressive at school. "Usually, Sammy can control his emotions, but he was so upset that we were gone for so long that he both purposefully and accidentally hurt several classmates," says Phyllis, who learned of the incidents only on the couple's return. "When we talked to him about it, he was upset with himself for losing control, but he was also able to tell us that he was angry at us for going away for so long. It will probably be a long time before we feel comfortable taking that long a vacation again," she adds.

If you suspect that your child may take out his frustration through misbehavior, talk to your caregiver, your child's teacher, and any other adult who may be in charge when the bad behavior occurs. It will be in your child's best interest to have them acknowledge that your child misses you and to channel his feelings in appropriate rather than hurtful ways.

TO CHECK IN . . . OR NOT?

When you're on a business trip, you will probably want to call home to be reassured that all's well and to hear about how your child's day has gone, from either your spouse, the caregiver, or your child herself. Keep in mind that no matter how much you would like to hear your child's voice, however, he may not necessarily feel the same way. Peggy Tabacco called home 2 hours after arriving in Palm Springs for a 48-hour weekend stay with her husband to let her parents, who were caring for their two children, know the number of the hotel they were staying at. "My son, Ted, got on the phone with me, asked me dozens of questions and then began lobbying for us to come back that night," says Peggy. She didn't call home again, and when she returned, her mother told her that Ted had been "down" for a long time after the call. "He had no problem saying goodbye to us, but hearing my voice so soon after we left disrupted the equilibrium he'd established without us," says Peggy. The next time she was away on a business trip, she avoided talking to her children until the night before she was due home. "It worked. Both of them were excited about telling me what they'd been doing with their dad in my absence, and Ted didn't have the same negative reaction," says Peggy. "The most important thing is to know your kid, which is usually accomplished on a trial-and-error basis," says child psychiatrist Dr. Julia Robertson. "Children are complicated and they change, so the best any parent who travels can do is to try to fine-tune your behavior each time until you learn what works best."

Of course, there's another problem with checking in: you may learn something that you'd prefer not to know until you get home because there's nothing you can do about it except worry. Ellen and Peter Comden (not their real names) went on a week-long vacation/business trip, a 7-hour-plane ride from their home, when their daughter, Alison, was 9 months old. Ellen's parents and sister helped out Ellen's regular caregiver. "When we got back, she had a bad case of intestinal flu," says Ellen. "I know she was angry with me for not being there when she needed me, but I couldn't have anticipated her illness, and I was glad that my parents didn't call me to say she was sick while I was gone."

If you are fairly confident that your child will be happy to hear from you (or your trip is a first and you need to find out), it's a good idea to arrange a time when you'll call in advance, so that your child or caregiver can be available. If your child is verbal but not skilled in communicating via telephone, keep your questions and statements simple. Ask how his pet cat is, whether he drew a picture at school, or whether he played with his best friend today. You might want to share a few details about your trip or your hotel with a 4- or 5-year old—such as that you could see snow on the mountains you flew over or that your room is high up on the thirty-fifth floor.

--------------------------------- ---------------------------------

Strategies for Staying in Touch

Here's a list of ideas for staying in touch to choose from; try the ones you find most appealing to find out if they provide comfort for your child.

* The day before you leave home, mail your preschool child a postcard; continue to send them frequently while you are away.
* Leave small, inexpensive presents—one for every day that you will be gone—for your child to open.
* Leave notes where your child will find them over a period of days.
* Tape record yourself reading some of your child's favorite stories.
* Buy a duplicate of your child's favorite book and read it to her over the telephone while she follows along in her own copy.
* Trade photos with your child—leave yours on the table beside his bed, and tell him that you will have his picture by your bed in your hotel.

--------------------------------- ✳ ---------------------------------

When Not to Go

If you have a choice about when to schedule a trip, it's better to plan it a time when you know things will be on an even keel for your child and there are no other major new things that he is having to adjust to. If your child is starting preschool the week before Labor Day weekend, don't make plans for just you and your spouse to get away that particular weekend. Instead, schedule it before school starts or several weeks later so that your child will have had a chance to acclimate. You should exercise the same kind of planning with other changes that may be major sources of stress to your child, including a move to a new house (even if you're just moving down the block), a change in sitters, the death of a pet, or grandparents who used to live nearby moving to a distant retirement community.

Traveling at a time when your child is sick or coming down with something is problematic because children of any age prefer to be in the comfort of their parents' arms when they're ill. But if the tickets are purchased and elaborate plans are in place, you'll have to make a judgment call about whether putting things off can be justified. Ann and Tom Carson faced that choice when they were a week away from starting a 2-week vacation to Europe. "We had successfully taken short trips, and felt that we needed more than two nights away to really wind down, so we made elaborate arrangements with a network of relatives and our regular caregiver," explains Ann. Their older daughter, who was then 2½, hadn't been able to shake a mysterious virus, and it wasn't until an hour before they left for the airport that hospital tests showed that nothing serious was wrong. "That, combined with having an uncle who was a pediatrician available in case anything further developed, gave us the peace of mind to go ahead with our plans," says Ann. "Our daughter got better, and both she and her younger sister did fine while we were gone."

Home Again

In many ways, the most important part of any separation is the reunion. You will no doubt fantasize about your child running, arms outstretched, to hug you as you walk off the plane, or having your parents place your blanketed babe into your arms and hearing her coo her delight that you've returned. But be forewarned: the reunion you fantasize may turn out quite differently.

Many children withdraw emotionally to protect themselves from missing a parent too much. Your baby may refuse to look you in the eye, your toddler may cling to your spouse or his caregiver, or your preschooler may continue the activity in which she's involved when you walk in the front door and may appear to be uninterested in your welcome. By acting detached instead of delighted, he is telling you in the best way he knows how that you are important to him, and that he is angry that you went away. Give him time to acclimate to your presence again. Don't insist on holding him or inserting yourself in the activity he's engaged in, but make yourself available, and try to get him to warm up to you. Say how much you missed him and how eager you are to see the art projects he worked on in your absence. Most children will be back in your arms within the hour, if not within minutes. But even if that's not the case, try to be understanding if the reaction goes on, even if it's for days.

When the Tells returned home after their 11-day vacation, their 4-year-old daughter Brette, who had been an angel in their absence, became very whiny and would have nothing to do with the grandparents who had been caring for her. "She didn't want to go to school, and she told us how sad she was while we were gone," says Phyllis. "It took about 5 days for Brette and her brother to begin feeling secure again and get back into their usual routine." It's not uncommon for older children to show their reactions to having been separated from you over the course of several days. And for some children, like Brette, acting good while you're gone or trying to be more loving than usual on your immediate return is a behavior designed to keep you from going away again. If that's the case, reassure her that nothing she did or did not do caused you to go away. Reiterate in terms she's likely to understand why Moms and Dads have to go on business trips or vacations. Another common reaction of children is their reluctance to let you out of their sight for a few days. To the extent that you can, just let your shadow follow you around or your clinging vine cling until he feels more confident that you aren't going to disappear again anytime soon.

Fathers who travel regularly on business often encounter a re-entry period when they return, as their spouse and child adjust to having them around again. "Jonathan, who is 6, is used to having more say around the house when his dad is gone," says Joan Harlem. "I'm more tolerant about the way things get done or don't get done than my husband Robert is, so when he comes home, Jonathan will often challenge his orders by saying, 'That's not how Mom and I do it,'" explains Joan. One of the strategies that Joan has used successfully to help Jonathan and her 4-year-old son get used to their dad again quickly is to disappear herself to run errands or visit a friend soon after Robert returns. "It seems that having him all to themselves helps break down the barriers of having been apart a little more quickly and re-establish their relationship again," says Joan.

WHEN YOUR KIDS GET THE GIMMES

As tempting as it may be to guarantee a smile on your child's face with a gift on your return, beware: if done regularly or to excess, it can interfere with the readjustment and bonding that have to happen once you're together again. "The gift you have brought home should not be a way of trying to buy off your child, to make him less upset about your being away," says Dr. Robertson. "What's more important is for you to be able to handle your child's being upset about your absence, and to help him learn how to express his feelings in an appropriate way. Let him know, for example, that you understand why he may not to interrupt what he's doing to talk to you right away, but hitting you is not acceptable," she adds.

On the other hand, gifts that help make where you went or what you did real to your child are fine. When Tom Schmidt travels on business, he tries to find just the right souvenirs, whether it's Gumby-like alligators from Florida or Wright brother–era model airplanes from North Carolina. Keep in mind that most kids are happy with trinkets, especially if they have the cachet of travel—little bags of peanuts from the airplane, tiny bottles of shampoo from the hotel, brochures or postcards showing pictures of the hotel where you stayed. If your child is 4 or older, make your gift part of a special ritual you share by starting a collection. Bring her charms for a bracelet to represent all the cities you visit, or T-shirts or caps with the logos of local sports teams.

If you or your spouse are traveling on business and don't anticipate having the time to go gift shopping, plan to do it in advance of your leaving. You might even want to leave the small surprise on your child's pillow the first night you're gone, or have your spouse plant it on the breakfast table the morning of your return. That way, you won't be bombarded with "What did you bring me?" the moment you walk in the door.

TRY, TRY AGAIN

Keep in mind that even when things don't go as well as you had hoped for you, your child, or the caregiver, you shouldn't rule out the possibility of trying again in the future. Says Dawn Basel, who tries to combine an annual vacation with her husband with one of her three required business trips each year: "You never stop missing your children, and you often feel guilty about leaving, but you learn through experience what makes it easier for all of you."

✿ SIX

Hospitalizations, Moves, and Military Duty

Every young child must experience normal separations, whether they involve Mom going to work, Dad going on a business trip, or the child going to daycare or school. But not every child must deal with traumatic separations and goodbyes that are the result of major illness, family relocations, or parental military duty. A University of London study found that children can be separated from their parents for quite long periods in early childhood with surprisingly little in the way of long-term effects. "The biggest fear for any child is the fear of abandonment," says Dr. Stana Paulauskas. "Whenever the separation from a parent is sudden, traumatic, or extended, that fear is likely to be activated unless the parent who is still at home doesn't try to hide the truth, even if it's a bad situation, and reassures the child that he or she will still be there for him," she says. In this chapter, you will find out how to minimize the distress that your child may feel when major, and sometimes unexpected, separations occur.

WHEN SICKNESS STRIKES

The need for hospitalization—yours or your child's—is among the most traumatic and painful of all types of separations. On top of whatever serious illness or injury necessitated the hospital stay, goodbyes—however short or temporary—are particularly difficult because of the stress everyone is feeling.

When a Parent Must Be Hospitalized

For young children, there are few things more difficult to understand than having Mom or Dad in the hospital. The most common reason for which a parent is hospitalized during a child's early years is when a sibling arrives. Going to the hospital to have a baby can be confusing; not only is your child losing you for a few days, but he may be fearful of what a new sister or brother might mean for him, so separation issues are likely to be intensified.

The good news is that pregnancies give you plenty of time to prepare your child for your hospitalization. Many hospitals now offer sibling classes for brothers- or sisters-to-be to tour the hospital with you and find out what to expect when the baby arrives. In a typical class, a film about what the child will see when he comes to visit you is shown, and the children get to see the maternity floor and the nursery. Children may be given lifelike dolls to hold for practice. "Hospitals can be overwhelming places for young children who come to visit a nursery after the birth of a sibling," says Kathleen McCue, M.A., L.S.W., supervisor of the Child Life Program at the Cleveland Clinic Foundation and president of the National Child Life Council, "so sneak previews can be useful in defusing a child's anxieties."

HANDLING A SCHEDULED HOSPITAL VISIT

If you know in advance that you or your spouse have to go into the hospital for an operation, it's important to be honest about where you are going and why. Inventing a story that you think will be less upsetting ("Mommy's going to be away on business for a few days") will backfire on you when your child figures out—as all but the very youngest child invariably will—where you really are. In addition to jeopardizing the trust he has in you, the story he pieces together to explain your hospital stay may actually be far worse than the truth. If you are going in for an appendectomy, for instance, you might say to your 3-year-old, "My tummy hurts right here, and it hurts so much that I need to go to the hospital where the doctors can make it feel better. When you see me, I'll have a big bandage on my tummy, like one I put on you when you have a boo-boo. I won't be able to pick you up for a week or two, but you can sit on the bed next to me so I can hug you."

HOW TO EXPLAIN A SUDDEN
HOSPITALIZATION TO A CHILD

When an accident or sudden illness occurs and a parent has to be hospitalized, there may be no time for a goodbye, but the well parent should try to explain what is going on to the child as soon as it's feasible. "Even if you're feeling overwhelmed by what's going on, making some kind of contact with your child is in her best interest," says McCue. "It's important to reassure your child that one of you is still okay."

Jenna McAllister (not her real name) was 5½ when her 41-year-old mother Beth suffered a ruptured aneurysm in her brain, which can be life-threatening. Beth was giving a business presentation when she suddenly felt her left side go numb. She was rushed to the hospital and spent the next month in the hospital.

Knowing what to say to your child when you're shell-shocked or unsure of the outcome is very difficult. "It's important to give your child information that is accurate but age appropriate," says McCue, "and if you can possibly talk to your child in person, it's better than a phone call."

"When Jenna asked where her mother was, I told her what had happened, and I also told her that Mom was going to get better," says Gary McAllister. "It's what I wanted to believe, and I decided that her only understanding of what was happening was going to be what I said, so I tried to be matter of fact but upbeat about it," he adds.

Gary did not give Jenna a detailed explanation of the circulatory system and what happens when an aneurysm bursts. Likewise, you need not share anatomical and medical information that will be more than your child can grasp or that may give her just enough information to invent a worse scenario than really exists.

Again, remember that toddlers and preschoolers are egocentric—they believe that everything that happens is connected with them. A 3-year-old, for instance, may sometimes believe that his own behavior somehow caused his mother or father to be ill or injured, so be sure to explain the why behind the accident or illness. "The bone in Daddy's leg broke when he fell off the ladder while he was painting your room this morning. It was just an accident and he's going to be fine very soon."

What's frightening to a child whose parent is unexpectedly absent is a departure from routine—being picked up by a relative or neighbor instead of a parent from school or daycare, for example, and not being told anything about what's going on. "Even a child under 6 months of age will react to a parent's unexpected absence," says Linda Goudas, Ph.D., staff psychologist at Children's Hospital in Boston. Infants can pick up on and be disturbed by changes in caregiving routine, which is why it's important for a parent who knows in advance that he or she is going to the hospital to say goodbye, however simply, or for the well parent to be as available as possible.

To Visit . . . or Not?

In most instances, children cannot stay with a parent who is in the hospital; some may even be restricted from visiting because of their age or the danger of being exposed to illness. If visiting is allowed, you need to think about—and perhaps talk with a patient representative about—whether it's in your child's best interest to see a hurt or sick parent and when. "In the event of a parent's unexpected hospitalization, it's important to assess how the child is faring with the separation," says McCue. "If he is eating and sleeping normally and is not feeling unusually sad or asking to see the sick parent, there's little point in taking the risk of him reacting badly to a hospital visit or his seeing a sick or hurt parent," she adds. An alternative to a hospital visit is sending home a photograph of the well parent standing next to the sick parent. "It allows you to explain where your spouse is, why he's there, and what the doctors are doing to help him get better," says McCue.

If you feel that your child can handle a visit to the hospital and very much wants to see the ill parent, try to prepare her for what she's going to see. Talk about the bandages that are swathed around Mommy's head or explain that the tubes that are going into Daddy's arm are delivering food, fluid, or medicine.

Gary McAllister decided that it would be best to delay Jenna's first trip to the hospital until Beth was out of intensive care. "Even though Jenna could not see her Mom for 6 days, it was better when they were finally reunited because some of the paralysis that had affected Beth's face had begun to dissipate, and she was sitting up in bed and could talk," says Gary.

Remember, too, that you cannot control what your child will see or hear in the corridors and elevators, and the smell of hospitals tends to be upsetting to children and adults alike (this is likely to be especially true if your child is easily overstimulated or reacts strongly to new experiences). Goudas advises parents to think about the timing of a hospital visit. "If in 12 or 24 hours the patient might be dramatically better, you should delay your visit," she says. If you have any doubts about whether a visit is wise, you can have your child talk to your spouse on the phone or have her keep in touch with Mommy or Daddy by drawing pictures that you can deliver.

Reassurances and Routine

If you or your spouse is in the hospital, one of the most difficult things for your child is that her life will be affected not only by the temporary loss of the sick parent but by the loss of the other parent's attention. "An adult's natural inclination is not to want to burden any one family member or friend, but to try to spread out the responsibility of caring for the child or children at home," says McCue. "But staying with Grandma on the weekend and Aunt Susie on Monday and Tuesday and going back home with a sitter on Wednesday is usually not in your child's best interest. She needs as much stability and routine as possible under these circumstances." The ideal solution is to arrange for a person or people your child knows and likes to come and stay in your home during the time of your spouse's hospitalization and recuperation.

Explain who will be taking care of her and how her days will be different or the same. You might say, for example, "You will still go to preschool and you will still ride home with Haley, and Grandma and Daddy will be here to take care of you when you get home.

But after supper, you all can come visit me in the hospital."

It's also smart to meet with your child's preschool or kindergarten teacher and any other adult with whom she spends regular time so that plans and expectations are understood by everyone else. "The teacher will be among the first to notice that your normally cheerful, outgoing child is a bit quiet or withdrawn, so it's essential for her to know what's going on," says McCue. If you want to maintain some privacy about details related to your spouse's medical condition, that's fine. You need share only facts that can help your caregiver or the teacher deal effectively with your child. The length of the hospital stay, the period of recuperation, whether or not the illness is life-threatening are all reasonable facts that should be shared.

About a week after her stroke, Beth McAllister was moved from an intensive-care ward to a rehabilitation ward, where things were looser. Says Gary, "Jenny and I soon settled into a routine. I took her to school, visited Beth in the hospital, went to work, picked Jenna up from school, and then we'd both go to the hospital to eat our evening meal together. Jenna adjusted quickly to this routine, which continued for several weeks. The fact that Beth was getting better and more animated helped. We all felt very lucky that while it had affected her physically (she had only minimal function in her left arm and leg), it hadn't affected her cognitively," he adds.

Beth came home for 6 days after her initial month's stay in the hospital. Then she returned to have three other detected aneurysms removed; although the surgery was successful, she gave everyone, including her surgeons, a scare when her condition deteriorated shortly thereafter. When she went home another 2½ weeks later, she was "drugged to the gills" and "non-functional," remembers Gary. "At that point so much of my energy and attention was focused on Beth that I didn't give much thought to Jenna's emotional well-being," says Gary, whose sister came to help him care for Jenna for several weeks. "It was after my sister left that Jenna began to complain that all I did was pay attention to Mom and not to her. That was probably true, so I tried to shift my focus. It got to the point where I could tell when she was feeling neglected because she'd act uncooperative about getting ready for school or just whine. Given the pressure of what was going on, those were good reminders for me," says Gary.

DELAYED REACTIONS

It's not uncommon for children to be themselves during the time a parent is hospitalized, but their ability to take events in stride may change at the time of the sick parent's homecoming. "Children will try to hold themselves together and be brave so that they can get through the time a parent is hospitalized," explains McCue, "but when the parent comes home and things have the potential to go back to normal, children often fall apart," she says.

The higher the level of stress in the family during the time of the parent's illness, the more pronounced a reaction you're likely to see. Your child may become angry at either the parent who became sick or had the

accident or the well parent whose energy was chan-
neled into keeping life as normal as possible. Another
possibility: your child may become withdrawn and reluctant to warm up to you, the sick parent, again. Or
she may become clingy and become upset if she
doesn't know where you are at all times.

All of these reactions are normal and are likely to
be short-lived if you and your spouse are able to give
your child time to adjust to new circumstances (your
being unable to do certain things, at least for a while)
and to re-establish routine in her life. It may, of course,
take months for life to return to anything remotely re-
sembling normal. Your child may lash out or become
frustrated when normalcy doesn't return quickly
enough.

Jenna McAllister would become angry with her
mother when she wasn't able to help Jenna open pack-
ages or help her with other tasks because her left arm
wasn't functioning well after her stroke. "One unrealis-
tic expectation I had of Jenna was for her to put her
mom ahead of herself," says Gary. "I'd tell her she
had to help out because there were some things Mom
couldn't do anymore. It was only later that I realized
how hard this must have been for a 6-year-old."

Anything that you and the sick parent can do to
help your child process what has happened and what
is likely to happen will help her. One effective tech-
nique that McCue suggests is to compose a storybook
about how the illness or accident has affected the family. Write simple sentences about what happened and
how it made you and your spouse and your child feel.
Cut out pictures from a magazine or draw stick figures
to accompany your words. The quality of the writing

and artwork isn't important; what does matter is that this homemade storybook give your child a concrete picture of what has happened. "If your child asks you to read it over and over again, you will know that he is trying to integrate the experience into his reality," says McCue. "If your child prefers reading his favorite storybooks, you'll know that he doesn't need this help right now," she adds. Keep the storybook open-ended so that you can add more experiences and feelings as needed.

Lots of reassurance that the sick parent is not going to vanish should help, too, and may be needed for weeks, if not months, depending on how sudden and traumatic the separation and illness or accident was.

When Your Child Must Be Hospitalized

Doctors and hospital administrators realize that children who are sick and separated from their parents are doubly stressed. "Separation from the parent during a hospitalization may be more traumatic for the child than the actual illness or injury," says Barry Zuckerman, M.D., a pediatrician at Boston City Hospital. Adds McCue, "What's more likely to upset a child is if her parents let their anxiety show, and that's more likely to happen if they don't understand the risks and the steps of the treatment."

Find out as much as you can in advance about what your child will experience, and prepare him in language he understands. Be honest—if there is going to be discomfort or pain, don't say that there won't be, or you will lose credibility with your child. For any admission that's not an emergency, find out whether the hospital has an orientation program for small children. At Yale–New Haven Hospital, for instance, parents and their children are given complete tours, including tours of the operating and recovery rooms for children scheduled for surgery. Procedures relevant to the child's condition are explained simply, honestly, and in child-appropriate language.

If your hospital has no such option, gather all the information you can beforehand. Talk with your pediatrician and ask what you and your child should expect. Get some children's books on what it's like to go to the hospital and read them together with your child. (See the Resource list at the end of this book for suggestions.)

If you know in advance that your child will have to be hospitalized, you can rehearse separation scenes. If your child is not used to routine separations, it can be as easy as your saying you're leaving the room, doing so, then coming back for increasingly longer increments of time. If your child has gone through routine separations with no problems, you may want to rehearse the specific separation that an operation, for example, will entail.

Most hospitals also allow parents to be with their children around the clock. Still, policies vary, and you may not be allowed to stay with your child at all times. That's why it's important for you and your child to develop a relationship with a child-life specialist, who can provide advice and support in your absence. If this type of professional is not available, ask a nurse or therapist you or your child likes if she can be with your child or available to your child when you cannot.

Be polite but persistent about your desire to stay

with your child whenever possible—digging in your heels as you smile often works surprisingly well. If your child must have surgery, for instance, ask if you can be with her until the anesthesia takes effect, and rejoin her as soon as she is brought into the recovery area so she won't be frightened if she awakens alone (many hospitals often allow this practice). "Parents know their child best, and how to comfort him or her," says M. G. Mendes de Leon, coordinator of the Child Life Program at Yale–New Haven Hospital in Connecticut. Enlist the support of your pediatrician in this cause—a word from her can sometimes work wonders.

Your job or need to be at home with your other children may mean that there will be times when you are away from your sick child's bedside. Even when you're at the hospital, your child may have to be alone for minutes or hours, so you can eat or go to the bathroom or speak with doctors. Whenever you must go, even if it's only for a few minutes, tell your child where you're going and when you will be back. "*Never* sneak out," says McCue. "It may hurt you less, but it's much harder for your child when she discovers that you're gone. And don't promise to return at a particular time unless you're certain you can be there," she adds.

Mendes de Leon suggests that if you need to leave for a few hours, start a task with your child that the two of you will finish when you return: read part of a story or begin a simple jigsaw puzzle. Tell your child, "I'm going to go home and check on your brothers, and Grandma will stay with you. When I come back, we'll finish the story together and find out how it ends."

If at all possible, try to arrange for someone the child knows and likes to be with him when you and your spouse cannot. "Some children are devastated when their parents have to leave, and even though hospital staff try to help them get through it, it would clearly be better for the child if someone else in their world can fill the gap," says McCue.

Once you made the decision to leave your child's bedside and you have done everything you can to make sure that he feels secure, including going through your goodbye ritual, go. If your child cries and you respond, he will use that tactic again to keep you by his bedside.

Finally, keep in mind that while being with your child as much as you can is a good idea, it's also important for you to get the rest you need (at home, if necessary) so that you have the energy you need to help your child cope with her recovery.

✳

When Your Child Is in the Hospital

- Have your child take her favorite toy or blanket to the hospital with her. Even an infant can be comforted with the familiar feel and smell of the quilt from his bed at home.
- Bring a framed photo of the family to put on the night stand by her bed. Pictures of pets are helpful, too.
- Ask the staff if your child can wear her own clothes. Even if she has to stay in bed, being able to wear her favorite pajamas and funny-face slippers can make things seem a little friendlier.

- Surprise your child with a special meal or two from home or her favorite take-out place if she's under no dietary restrictions.

- When you must leave her bedside, tell your child exactly where you are going and when you will be back.

- Share the bedside watch with your spouse or another relative or close friend so that you can eat and sleep properly; you'll be a much bigger help and comfort to your child if you're mentally alert.

- Ask if one or two regular nurses can be assigned to your child so that he isn't experiencing a constant stream of new faces (a policy that's standard practice in some hospitals). A child of about 3 or older should be shown how to work the call button to ask for what he needs if you are not there.

- If your child has to endure uncomfortable tests or procedures, ask if she can bring her favorite doll or stuffed animal along. Some hospitals even allow such objects to accompany children into the operating room.

- Hang up drawings your child has done near your child's bed (if possible) so that the staff who cares for him will see him as an imaginative individual and treat him that way, especially if his illness or injury makes that difficult.

IMPACT OF GEOGRAPHIC MOVES

Children can experience separation anxiety if you make a move that means they must say goodbye to everything that's become familiar to them in their young lives. Preparing young children for how a relocation will affect them is a smart idea. Showing them photographs of the new house and backyard, a nearby playground or park area, or even the resident llama at a local petting zoo can help make the future more real to them. Talk about why you're making the move—a new and better job for Mom or Dad, the proximity to friends or family (and what that will mean in terms of how often they can visit or spend time with them), or the bigger, nicer house and backyard they'll have.

"Children will copy you, so if you are upbeat and comfortable about the move, the child is likely to see it as an exciting new adventure, too," says Dr. Carol Seefeldt. "If, however, you are anxious or fearful about the relocation, your child is likely to feel that way, too," she says. You shouldn't avoid talking about the sad things connected with your move—having to say goodbye to friends or family, not being able to go back to a preschool or daycare situation your child loves, or having to part with a pet who cannot come along. "Acknowledge your feelings or your child's, but then focus on the future and, if it makes sense, suggest how you can deal with the sadness," says Dr. Seefeldt— "for example, by 'adopting' a grandmother in your new location."

Even when you try to ensure smooth sailing, however, your child may react by acting out his feelings to being in new situations. Peggy and Joe Tabacco knew that their cross-country move from New York to California was going to be a big one for them and their two children, Ted, who had just turned 5, and Christina, who was 3½. "We felt very positive about the move because it was one that we both chose to make based on a 3-month experimental stay that was related to my husband's work," explains Peggy. "We decided that it was a now-or-never proposition because it would only be harder to do once the kids started school. And although we weren't leaving any relatives who lived anywhere nearby, we all had to say goodbye to friends who were a very important part of our daily lives," she says.

Ted and Christina seemed to think of the move as the great adventure their parents did as they watched the big moving van pull away with all their belongings. They had a great goodbye barbecue with their closest friends, followed by a family reunion before they headed to their new home. But 2 days after they arrived, school started, and so did Ted's protests. He did not want to go to kindergarten, even though he had 2 years of preschool under his belt. "Every day, our fight escalated," remembers Peggy. "About 2 weeks into the school year, I told him that he had to walk from the drop-off gate to his classroom by himself, although I would walk along on the other side of the fence most of the way. As we walked, he screamed at me, 'You're the meanest mom in the world. I hate you for making me do this!' I went home with my stomach in knots," she says. When Ted finally adopted the strategy of attaching himself to her leg as she walked him into class, Peggy took the teacher up on her suggestion: Ted could go back home, but he had to sit in a room with no toys, TV, or books until the hour that school ended. The strategy worked; about 10 minutes into his first dull day at home, Ted asked his mother to walk him back to school.

"I realized that Ted's school goodbye problems were related to our move, that having to get used to a new teacher and a new school on top of a different house and a different way of life (they'd moved from Manhattan to a suburban area) was the final straw," says Peggy. "It was his way of saying 'This is really hard for me.'" To try to get him acclimated as quickly as possible, Peggy orchestrated playdates with classmates several times a week. "It not only helped him, it helped me because I got to know the parents of his classmates much more quickly, and several of them became good friends," she says. As is often the case, Ted's sister didn't have the same reaction. "She went to her new preschool without a complaint, but even at that age, it was clear to me that she had the kind of temperament that made her more independent and better able to cope with change than was Ted," says Peggy.

Coping with a Series of Moves

No matter how well you think you know your child, it's usually impossible to foresee what the consequences of a big move are likely to be. And young children are not always willing to accept or capable of accepting all the adult reasons for why a move has to happen. The Higleys found themselves faced with some extremely difficult situations when they made a series of geographic moves between their daughter's fourth and sixth birthdays.

When Sally was four, Scott and Julie Higley (not their real names) moved to Manhattan from London because Julie was offered a job by her company that was too good to turn down. Scott and Julie were returning to a place where they'd both lived for over a decade. But Sally knew only London, where she had been born. In the months preceding the move, Julie traveled frequently between New York and London to hammer out the details of the new job. Often, she had to delay coming home for several days. "Although I worked from home and was helping Sally's nanny take care of her, Sally would inevitably get upset when I told her Mommy wasn't coming back on the original day. Sometimes she cried. Sometimes she got angry and misbehaved. And she began having problems falling asleep at night," remembers Scott, a free-lance newspaper correspondent.

Once the Higleys settled into life in New York, Sally's sleeping problems got worse. "It got to the point that she could not go to sleep unless one of us stayed with her," says Scott, "and she would often wake at night and crawl into bed with us or want one of us to come sleep with her. And that had not happened before." But Sally adjusted to school and began to spend a lot of time with children whose parents were close friends of her own parents.

But 20 months into her new life in the United States, Sally's parents moved to a weekend home they owned when Julie's job situation suddenly changed. Even though Sally had spent a lot of weekends at this house, moving there was the third move since the family had come back to the United States. (After 8 months in their first sublet apartment, the owners returned, and the Higleys had to move into another sublet.) And Sally, who was almost 6, began attending her third new school. "It was a difficult time in our lives, and Sally reacted. When we put her down at night, she wanted the TV on or for us to talk so that she could hear us. She told us the dark and the quiet scared her. And she always wanted to know where one or the other of us was; we couldn't leave her alone in a room," remembers Scott.

Luckily, Sally's love affair with school continued, and her teacher made a particular effort to make her feel at home. Five months later, the Higleys decided to move back to London to accept a new offer from Julie's employer. "We had mixed feelings about the move, and Sally picked up on that. She also reacted negatively because I had been a stay-at-home mom for the previous 6 months, and now that we were going back to London, she'd knew I'd be back at work," says Julie.

This last move proved to be the most difficult of all for Sally. She was behind academically in school, so the one thing she'd always been able to count on—being at the head of her class—was gone. There were times during the first few weeks that the Higleys thought they should pack their bags and go back to the United States.

A year after their move back to London, her parents reported that Sally was thriving, doing well in school, and being affectionate in the way that a secure child is. "Scott and I really went to great lengths to reassure Sally that life isn't one big goodbye, that friends will always be friends even if they move away, and that most importantly, home is wherever the three of us are," says Julie.

Regressions and Behavioral Problems

If, after a move, your child experiences eating, sleeping or goodbye problems or regressive behavior, it's a good idea to try to figure out what is bothering her, suggests Dr. Julia Robertson. "It may be a specific problem that has come up rather than moving itself," she says.

One important area to explore is what important people in your child's life were left behind. "The loss of a person your child was close to can be as traumatic for her as the death of that person would be," says Dr. Robertson. For many young children, that special person is the nanny or caregiver. "The fact that this person disappears from her life, and that there's no foreseeable time that the child will see them again, is a very difficult thing for a child to process," says Dr. Robertson.

If you suspect that saying goodbye to a caregiver or a special friend may be the source of your child's stress, try to talk to her about it. Again, keep in mind that children often do not respond to direct questions; you may have to get at the issue through play. "Children who are preoccupied with something are likely to bring it up in play," says Dr. Robertson. (See the Resources section to get information on a video explaining "floor time," a concept developed by Stanley Greenspan, M.D., that explains how you can better identify and understand your child's feelings through play.) Acknowledge your child's feelings of sadness and loss by saying, for example, "I miss Jade, too. She was a great babysitter and friend. But she couldn't come with us because she needed to live near her own family." Says Dr. Seefeldt, "And, of course, do a lot of comforting and holding and assuring the child that everything will work out."

If sleep problems arise in response to such a problem or simply because your child is fearful of the different noises or look of his room at night, try what psychologists call successive approximation to curb the undesirable behavior. In the case of a child like Sally who cannot go to sleep or insists on coming into your bed, for example, you will want to take steps each night to get her back into her normal routine. Allow the things that your child asks for that aren't a big deal: leaving even a bright light on (and perhaps dimming it or settling for less bright lights each successive night), allowing a radio or TV to be on (and turning down the volume each night), allowing all your child's stuffed animals in her bed, instead of just her one favorite one. If your child begs to sleep in your bed, offer to do something that will allow everyone to sleep better and is less likely to develop into a bad habit. Do what you're comfortable with and feel will work for your child: offer to take her back into her room and tuck her in, or stay in bed with him until he falls asleep, or allow him to sleep in a sleeping bag at the foot of your bed, at least for 1 or 2 nights (or move a few feet closer to his own room in it each night). "The important thing is to not let the behavior get out of hand," says Dr. Seefeldt. "All children want their parents to set limits; in the end, that's what makes them feel safe and taken care of."

WHEN UNCLE SAM CALLS

Being apart from one or both parents is easier for children to handle if they know when Mom or Dad is leaving and coming back, but that kind of predictability isn't always the case when one of you belongs to the armed forces. You may be assigned a tour of duty that doesn't include family or, worse yet, sent to a troubled part of the world. The uncertainty of when or even if things will return to normal can make a child's life very difficult. And the parent who has to cope with a spouse's illness or absence has to deal with both the child's anxiety and his or her own.

Chris Heffelfinger was a lawyer in private practice when he got orders to report for duty as a Marine Corps Reserve officer as part of Operation Desert Storm in December 1990. He left behind his 3-year-old son Jamie and his wife Marcia. "I had known that he was on alert since August," says Marcia, who was going through a difficult second pregnancy. "The day he got his orders, on December 1, I had a miscarriage," she says. When it came time for Chris to leave, he told his son: "Daddy doesn't want to go, but he has to. I'll come back, but I'm not sure just when." Marcia and Jamie had a very lonely Christmas. "We went through the motions of the holidays, but I was in a daze," she says.

Marcia describes her son as shy and reserved by nature; during his father's absence, Jamie became even more withdrawn. At preschool, he would take a big black crayon and scribble angrily. Jamie did not say anything about his father's absence for several months. Then one day when he and his mom were out walking their dog, he announced out of the blue: "Mommy, when I grow up, I'm never going to join the army and leave you."

How to Explain a Military Absence

To help your child cope when you must be away in a service-related capacity, be as honest as possible and use language that she can understand. Talk about where you are going and for how long. If you don't know when you will be returning, say so, but emphasize that you will be back as quickly as you are able. With a child under 4, this point is well worth emphasizing. Since young children tend to view the world as if it revolves around them, they tend to explain events in terms of their own involvement. Make sure your child knows that it is not because of him that you are going away, but because your job requires you to.

It is important for young children to feel that you are accessible. If you can be reached by phone, tell your child that, explaining that "Daddy (or Mommy) knows how to call me while I'm away working." If you are not going to be accessible by phone, ask your child to draw pictures or dictate notes for you while you are gone, and ask your spouse to send them to you. If your absence will be longer than a week, write to your child whenever possible, even if only to drop a brief note telling him something funny you saw that day, or just that you love and miss him. Chris Heffelfinger made tapes of himself reading his son's favorite stories before he left the country, and made several more while he was gone. "Jamie loved listening to those tapes," says Marcia. "It really comforted him to hear his father's voice."

If there is the potential for danger in your deployment, should you be frank about this with your child? Although you must be truthful with your child, it is probably best to not volunteer this kind of information and to be reassuring about how you answer your child's questions about possible dangers. "You have to be optimistic, not realistic with a young child," says Frederic J. Medway, Ph.D., professor of psychology at the University of South Carolina in Columbia. "You can never say there's a chance you might die, because your child will not only worry but may become dysfunctional, so that when you come back, she may have difficulty accepting your return because she has already prepared herself for the worst," he says. If your child asks directly whether you might be hurt, be honest but upbeat: "There might be some fighting where I am going, but my job has trained me to be very careful and to keep myself safe when I'm working."

Marcia Heffelfinger was careful not to let her son watch television news while his father was away in case he saw and was frightened by news covered by events there. But on a trip to the emergency room to repair a chin injury, Jamie saw footage of soldiers wearing gas masks. "I started crying, but Jamie didn't react," she says. "But then when Chris next called, Jamie said, 'Hi, Daddy. Are you wearing a gas mask?'" Fortunately, the war ended before Chris's unit was sent to conduct house-to-house combat in Kuwait City, the mission for which they were training. Dr. Martha Cox says, "When a parent is going into a potentially dangerous situation, it's best not to share your fears, but you must allow your child to feel and express his feelings and not deny to yourself the possibility that he may not be fearful simply because he is a child."

The Happiness and Stress of a Reunion

The most difficult part of a military-related separation may be your reunion with your child. Your child may be angry and withdrawn and require a great deal of reassurance in word and deed from you and your spouse before he can feel comfortable again. Or he may not show his feelings, but his behavior may indicate a continuing level of apprehension about losing you again. "Even though Jamie warmed up to Chris right away when he returned, it took Jamie several weeks to feel really relaxed again; he really held his feelings in. My mother-in-law used to say, 'I wish he'd have a temper tantrum or something!'" says Marcia Heffelfinger.

What you can do to help your child release his feelings in a positive way is to talk about your feelings so that he knows it's okay to express them. You might say, "I'm really happy that Daddy is back, but even now I sometimes find myself feeling sad that he missed your birthday. The good news is that he won't be going away again for a long time."

"The literature is clear that kids' reactions to a homecoming often mirror the reaction of the parents," says Dr. Medway. "If a man has been away for a while, whether it's because of military duty or because of frequent business trips, women don't always want to relinquish the role they've played as head of the household. And that can cause arguments and raise the level of tension in the house," he adds. If you have conflicts that have to be resolved with a spouse, it's important to avoid showing or voicing your feelings to or in front of your child. Instead, talk to your spouse, or, if necessary, talk to a professional about the difficulty you're having with your spouse's re-entry into your life.

ADJUSTMENT THROUGH TIME OR WITH HELP?

Keep in mind that your child may require time to adjust to new circumstances whenever a major illness, move, or separation occurs. Given your own emotional overload, tuning in to what's going on with your child may require more effort on your part. If his behavior, words, or actions indicate that he's having a hard time and the suggestions that have been made throughout this book don't seem to be making a difference, don't be afraid to seek out the help of a professional (see page 59 in Chapter Two for specific recommendations). Finding an objective, trained person who can help you navigate through difficult transitions will probably provide the relief and remedies your family needs.

Final Thoughts

By the time your child is old enough for first grade, you will have weathered hundreds, if not thousands, of separations. Some will have been so trivial you will no longer remember them, and neither will your child. Others will never be forgotten by either of you. But each separation, from the first time your baby cried when you went briefly to another room, to the day the two of you parted at the schoolroom door, is important. And each goodbye teaches a lesson about trust.

The separations of the early years provide the most basic opportunities for your child to learn how to handle separations throughout life. They also provide your child with practice in making transitions from one loved caregiver to another, in taking care of his own emotional needs until he is reunited with you, and in communicating his needs to important people other than you.

This book discusses many different types of situations in which you are likely to take leave of your child. Here, once again, are the basics to keep in mind whether your separation is a routine one, or one that's out of the ordinary. If you follow these guidelines, know that your child will develop the kind of secure attachment to you that's critical to future, happy goodbyes.

- Find the best, most reliable caregiver you can.
- Disrupt the child's normal routine as little as possible.
- Be honest about the nature and expected length of the separation.
- Return when you say you are going to.
- Take your child's developmental level into account.
- Consider your child's temperament.
- Acknowledge your child's feelings about separations.
- Never leave without saying goodbye.

While it is normal for all children to prefer to stay with their families from time to time, if your child reaches his late preschool or early school years and regularly has trouble separating from you, however, it's in your child's and your own best interest to get professional help. The following behaviors are indicative of problems that are in your child's best interest to address:

- He consistently refuses social invitations like parties or outings with friends, always preferring to stay home with you.

- She used to separate without difficulty, but has begun to resist separations again.
- He is extremely vigilant about your comings and goings and worries excessively when you leave his side or his sight.
- Routine separations make her cry or throw tantrums.
- He has been asked to leave a preschool program or daycare setting because his separation difficulties were persistent or too disruptive.
- She is with you so constantly that you are feeling trapped and resentful.
- He continues to articulate fears that you or your spouse will die, long after an illness has been successfully treated.

Realize that as your child grows, separations will differ from those of early childhood in important respects. For one thing, the number of separations precipitated by your needs (going to work, attending a meeting, going to a doctor's appointment) versus those precipitated by your child's schedule (school, a birthday party, team practice) will just about balance out. The older your child gets, the more occasions there are in his life that require him to separate from you. The social pull of his world will grow greater with every year, so that "No, Mom, please don't go" becomes "Oh, Mom, please can I go?" with amazing speed. From time to time, you may be left feeling as bewildered and, yes, even a little abandoned, as he was as a toddler waving goodbye to you.

Resources

BOOKS

Balaban, Nancy. *Learning to Say Goodbye: Starting School and Other Early Childhood Separations.* Signet, 1987 (out of print but available in some libraries)

Belsky, Jay. *The Transition to Parenthood.* Dell Publishing, 1995

Brenner, Barbara. *The Preschool Handbook: Making the Most of Your Child's Education.* Pantheon, 1990

Garber, Stephen W., Garber, Marianne Daniels, and Spizman, Robin Freedman. *Monsters Under the Bed and Other Childhood Fears.* Villard Books, 1993

Jervis, Kathe. *Separation: Strategies for Helping Two to Four Year Olds.* National Association for the Education of Young Children, 1992

Lieberman, Alicia. *The Emotional Life of the Toddler.* The Free Press, 1994

McCue, Kathleen. *How to Help Children Through a Parent's Serious Illness.* St. Martins Press, 1994

Weisberg, Anne C., and Bucker, Carol A. *Everything a Working Mother Needs to Know*. Doubleday, 1994

Zigler, Edward F., and Lang, Mary E. *Child Care Choices*. The Free Press, 1991

VIDEO

Floor Time: Tuning Into Each Child. Scholastic Incorporated, Early Childhood Division, 730 Broadway, New York, NY 10003. $74.95

ARTICLES

Block, Michele. "Suddenly It's Cling Time." *Parents*, June, 1993

Borden, Marian Edelman. "Parents' Night Out." *American Baby*, November, 1994

Brown, Carol Deasy. "Sitting Pretty." *Parenting*, February, 1993

Cadden, Vivian. "How Kids Benefit From Child Care." *Working Mother*, April, 1994

Cassidy, Anne. "From Home to Day Care: How to Make Goodbyes and Hellos Easier." *Parents*, November, 1994

Cassidy, Anne. "What Scares Toddlers." *Parents*, June, 1994

Cushman, Kathleen, and La Farge, Phyllis. "Off to a Great Start: Preparing Children for Preschool." *Parents*, October, 1992

Eastman, P. "Kids! Birth to 2" (routines and sleep; easing separation anxiety). *Working Mother*, March, 1994

Gibson, Debra. "Battling the Bye-Bye Blues." *Better Homes and Gardens*, September, 1994

Greenspan, Stanley. "The Preschool Transition: Tune in to Your Child's Needs and Guarantee Her an Easy Adjustment." *Parents*, September, 1994

Karges-Bone, Linda. "How to Deal with Separation Anxiety." *American Baby*, August, 1994

Kemp, Theresa, and Gardephe, Colleen. "When One Spouse Travels." *Parents*, November, 1994

Kutner, Lawrence. "When Your Child Is Hospitalized." *Parents*, April, 1992

Leonard, June. "Morning Madness: How Working Parents Get Their Children Ready For School." *Redbook*, September, 1992

Levine, James A., Ed. "The Frequent Flyer Dad." *Child*, March, 1995

Levine, Karen. "When You Have to Travel." *Parents*, February, 1993

Maxey, Gabrielle. "Babysitting Co-ops." *American Baby*, April, 1992

McGinnis, Christopher. "Family Leave: How to Be There for Your Kids When Business Takes You Away." *Entrepreneur*, July, 1994

Meyer, Judith. "Your Child's Hospital Stay." *Parents*, April, 1994

Newman, Judith. "What Your Babysitter Wants You to Know." *Parenting*, March, 1994

Satran, Pamela Redmond. "In Search of the Perfect Sitter." *Working Mother*, July, 1993

Stern, Ellen Sue. "It's Tough to Leave the Baby." *American Baby*, January, 1994

Stern, Ellen Sue. "Day Care Guilt." *American Baby*, November, 1993

Weissbourd, Bernice. "Mommy, Please Don't Go." *Parents*, September, 1992

Weissbourd, Bernice. "How to Choose a Caregiver." *Parents*, August, 1992

Wilson, Donald. "Leaving Home Without Them." *Parenting*, February, 1992

Wingate, Carrie. "Starting Day Care." *American Baby*, November, 1994

Winn, Steven. "With Reservations." *Parenting*, February, 1994

Wise, Nicole. "Parting Is Such Sweet Sorrow." *Parenting*, June–July 1994

BOOKS TO SHARE WITH YOUR CHILD

Ackerman, Karen. *By the Dawn's Early Light*. Atheneum, 1994 (Two children stay with their grandmother when their mom works at night.)

Alda, Arlene. *Sonya's Mommy Works*. Little Simon, 1982

Anderson, Peggy Perry. *Time for Bed, the Babysitter Said*. Houghton Mifflin, 1987

Asch, F. *Goodbye, House*. Prentice-Hall, 1986

Bauer, Caroline Feller. *My Mom Travels a Lot*. Puffin Books, 1985

Berenstain, Stan and Jan. *Mama's New Job*. Random House, 1984

Blaine, Marge. *The Terrible Thing That Happened at Our House*. Four Winds Press, 1980 (Mom goes to work and the family solves related problems.)

Breinberg, Petronella. *Shawn Goes to School*. Crowell, 1974

Bucknall, Caroline. *One Bear in the Hospital*. Dial Books, 1984

Crary, Elizabeth. *Mommy Don't Go*. Parenting Press, 1986

de Regniers, Beatrice Schenk. *Waiting for Mama*. Clarion, 1984

Eisenberg, Phyllis Rose. *You're My Nikki*. Dial Books for Young Readers, 1992 (Nikki wants to be sure her mom won't forget her when she's working.)

Fowler, Susi L. *I'll See You When the Moon Is Full*. Greenwillow Books, 1994 (Dad goes on a two-week business trip.)

Hautzig, Deborah. *A Visit to the Sesame Street Hospital*. Random House, 1985

Hellard, Susan. *Eleanor and the Babysitter*. Little, Brown, 1991

Honeycutt, Natalie. *Whistle Home*. Orchard Books, 1993 (Mama goes to town for the day.)

Howe, James. *The Hospital Book*. Crown, 1984

Hutchins, Pat. *Three-Star Billy*. Greenwillow Books, 1994 (Billy is a monster who doesn't want to be in nursery school.)

McKinley, Robin. *My Father Is in the Navy*. Greenwillow Books, 1992 (A girl doesn't remember her father, who has been away at sea.)

Miranda, Anne. *Baby-sit*. Joy Street, 1990

Oxenbury, Helen. *First Day of School*. Dial Books for Young Readers, 1983 (A little girl goes to nursery school.)

Rey, Margret. *Curious George Goes to the Hospital*. Houghton Mifflin, 1966

Rockwell, Anne F. *My Baby-Sitter*. Collier Macmillan, 1985

Rogers, Fred. *Going to the Hospital*. Putnam, 1988

Rogers, Fred. *Going to Day Care*. Putnam, 1985

Rogers, Fred. *Moving*. Putnam, 1987

Smith, Lucia B. *My Mom Got a Job*. Holt, Rinehart and Winston, 1979

Stecher, Miriam B. *Daddy and Ben Together*. Lee & Shepard Books, 1981 (Mommy goes on a business trip.)

Viorst, Judith. *The Good-Bye Book*. Atheneum, 1988 (Child protests parents going out for the evening.)

Waber, Bernard. *Ira Says Goodbye*. Houghton Mifflin, 1988 (Saying goodbye to a best friend who is moving.)

Warren, Cathy. *Fred's First Day*. Lothrop, Lee & Shepard Books, 1984

Waggoner, Karen. *The Lemonade Babysitter*. Little, Brown, 1992

Ziefert, Harriet. *Harry Gets Ready for School*. Puffin, 1991

ORGANIZATIONS

Many professional organizations provide information or services that may be of help to parents.

American Academy of Pediatrics
P.O. Box 927
Elk Grove Village, IL 60009-0927
(800) 433-9016

The AAP offers brochures on a variety of topics of interest to parents, including selecting daycare and starting preschool.

American Council of Nanny Schools
Delta College, Room A-67
University Center, MI 48710
(517) 686-9417

This association of accredited nanny schools maintains a registry of graduates from accredited programs.

Au Pair in America
American Institute for Foreign Study
102 Greenwich Avenue
Greenwich, CN 06830
(800) 727-2437 or (203) 869-9090

The nation's oldest and largest au pair organization matches au pairs with families on a year-long or summer-long program. Au pairs come in on visas, and no taxes must be paid to the government by the host family.

Child Care Action Campaign
330 7th Avenue
New York, NY 10001
(800) 424-2246

CCAC provides information for parents seeking child care.

Child Care Aware
National Association of Child Care Resource and Referral Agencies
1319 F. Street, N.W., Suite 606
Washington, D.C. 20004
(800) 424-2246

This toll-free hotline can put you in touch with licensed caregivers and centers in your area.

National Association for the Education of Young Children (NAEYC)
Box 518, 1509 16th Street, N.W.
Washington, D.C. 20036
(800) 424-2460

Send a self-addressed, stamped envelope for their brochure on finding infant and toddler daycare. The association can also provide information about programs in your area that are accredited by NAEYC.

NAEYC also publishes "So Many Goodbyes: Ways to Ease the Transition Between Home and Groups Between Young Children," by Janet Brown McCracken.

About the Authors

Nancy Hall, M.S., M.Phil., is a developmental psychologist and a consultant with the Yale University Bush Center in Child Development and Social Policy. A former preschool teacher, she is a frequent contributor to *Child* and other parenting magazines, and the coauthor of *Children, Families and Government: Preparing for the 21st Century*. She lives in southern Connecticut with her husband, son, and daughter.

Peggy Schmidt has written hundreds of articles on parenting, education, and job-search strategies for national publications, including *The New York Times, Child, Working Woman, Glamour, First for Women,* and *New Woman*. Her syndicated column, "Your New Job," has been carried in the (New York) *Daily News,* the *Boston Herald,* the *Oakland Tribune,* and the *Atlanta Journal-Constitution*. She has taught feature writing to journalism undergraduates at New York

University and served as career coordinator for the New York University Summer Publishing Institute for 6 years. Her books include *The Job Hunter's Catalog* (John Wiley & Sons); *The 90 Minute Resume* (Peterson's); *Making It Big in the City: A Woman's Guide to Living, Loving and Working There* (McGraw Hill); and *Making It On Your First Job* (Avon Books). She currently serves as West Coast director of the American Book Producers Association and as program chair of the Electronic Publishing special interest group of the San Francisco chapter of the International Interactive Communication Society.

She lives with her husband and two young children in Portola Valley, California.

child

The magazine for today's parents

New solutions, fresh ideas, expert advice, good old common sense and the experiences of people like you who are raising kids in the real world. Read it first in child.

YES!

Send me a free issue of child.

If I like it I'll receive a one year subscription (10 issues in all, including my free issue) for just $8.97 — a savings of over 69% off newsstand. If I choose not to subscribe, I simply return the bill marked "cancel." The free issue is mine to keep.

To order call 1-800-777-0222 extension 1122
Rate good in U.S. only

....

Look for all the helpful books in the child magazine series

SLEEP
TANTRUMS
GOODBYES

Available from Pocket Books

POCKET
B O O K S

1220